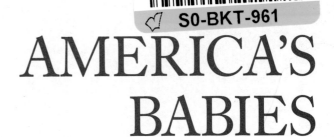
SO-BKT-961

AMERICA'S BABIES

The ZERO TO THREE Policy Center

DATA BOOK

By CINDY OSER AND JULIE COHEN

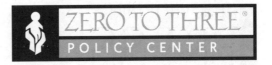

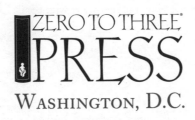

ZERO TO THREE
PRESS
WASHINGTON, D.C.

CHABOT COLLEGE LIBRARY

REF
HQ
774.5
.O75
2003

▌ZERO TO THREE
▌PRESS

Published by
ZERO TO THREE
2000 M St., NW, Suite 200
Washington, DC 20036-3307
(202) 638-1144
Toll-free orders (800) 899-4301
Fax: (202) 638-0851
Web: http://www.zerotothree.org

Cover and text design: Touch 3, Art Director Vanessa Sifford

Copyright 2003 by ZERO TO THREE. All rights reserved.
For permission for academic photocopying (for course packets, study materials, etc.) by copy centers, educators, or university bookstores or libraries, of this and other ZERO TO THREE materials,
please contact Copyright Clearance Center, 222 Rosewood Drive, Danvers, MA 01923; phone,
(978) 750-8400; fax, (978) 750-4744; or visit its Web site at www.copyright.com.

First Edition First Printing October 2003
ISBN 0-943657-66-0
Printed in the United States of America

Suggested citation:
Oser, C., & Cohen, J. (2003). *America's babies: The ZERO TO THREE Policy Center data book.*
Washington, DC: ZERO TO THREE Press.

TABLE OF CONTENTS

LIST OF FIGURES AND TABLES

PREFACE

From the time they are born until they arrive at the school house door, young children in America are largely ignored by public and private policymakers. And yet, we know from the science of early childhood development that babies and toddlers cannot wait. These earliest days, months, and years of life are ones of incredible vulnerability as well as promise. It is during this time that the brain undergoes its most dramatic development and children acquire the ability to think, speak, learn, and reason.

Babies are born ready to learn. Positive experiences and nurturing, responsive relationships with parents and other important caregivers support children's healthy growth and development. Research shows that early experiences and warm, loving relationships form "both the foundation and the scaffold on which cognitive, linguistic, emotional, social, and moral development unfold" (Shonkoff & Phillips, 2000, p. 349). Research also shows that when experiences fail to support a baby or toddler's biologically inherent desire to learn, grow, and succeed, "a child's motivation diminishes, shifts, or finds problematic outlets" (Shonkoff & Phillips, 2000, p. 32).

The purpose of *America's Babies: The ZERO TO THREE Policy Center Data Book* is to paint a portrait of the lives of babies and toddlers in our nation. We wanted this book to provide as complete a picture as possible. Yet, the picture we present is far from complete. Why? Many basic facts have not been collected, and in many areas the data simply do not exist. We cannot report, for example, the status of mental health and social–emotional development in infants and toddlers. We do not know how many infants and toddlers are waiting for child care or how many infants and toddlers are witnessing domestic violence on a regular basis. Why don't we know how many fathers are present at the birth of their babies? As we researched and prepared this book, we often asked: Why do these data not exist? Why have planners, policy shapers, and decision makers not asked the questions we have asked? Sadly, we can only conclude this is symptomatic of the largely invisible nature of babies and young children in our society.

America's Babies presents facts and figures, not policy alternatives. This is not to say that we do not know how to address the needs of infants, toddlers, and families. We do. That is why we created the ZERO TO THREE Policy Center. The Center brings the voice of babies and toddlers to public policy at the federal, state, and local levels. We translate scientific research into language that is accessible and useful for policymakers. We cultivate leadership for babies and toddlers in states and communities. We study and share promising state and community strategies for promoting the healthy growth and development of babies and toddlers. Look to us at www.zerotothree.org/policy as a resource in your own work.

We hope this book will lead to the creation of more champions for America's babies. As a nation we can, and must, do more to help families and communities do the best by their babies. One day we will all need them as much as they need us now. Our destinies are intertwined. Our future is their future. Our babies are waiting.

Sheila B. Kamerman, D.S.W.
Co-Chair, ZERO TO THREE
Legislative Task Force
Compton Foundation Centennial Professor
Columbia University School of Social Work

J. Ronald Lally, Ed.D.
Co-Chair, ZERO TO THREE
Legislative Task Force
Director, Center for Child &
Family Studies, WestEd

Matthew E. Melmed
Executive Director
ZERO TO THREE

Erica Lurie-Hurvitz
Director
ZERO TO THREE Policy Center

ACKNOWLEDGMENTS

ZERO TO THREE acknowledges the significant efforts of Tim Champney, Ph.D., and Frank Funderburk, Ph.D., from the Delmarva Foundation for Medical Care in collecting and analyzing data for this book. In addition, we thank Dana Chieco and Jodi Jacobson Chernoff, Ph.D., for their diligent attention to detail, and Judith Jerald, Early Head Start Coordinator, Head Start Bureau; Barbara A. Thompson, Office of Children and Youth, Department of Defense; George L. Askew, M.D.; Joan Lombardi, Ph.D.; Joy Osofsky, Ph.D.; Kyle Pruett, M.D.; and Fred Wulczyn, Ph.D., Research Fellow, Chapin Hall Center for Children, University of Chicago.

We also wish to thank members of the ZERO TO THREE Policy Task Force for their time and advice: Carol Berman, Ph.D., Linda Gilkerson, Ph.D., Sheila Kamerman, D.S.W., Ronald Lally, Ed.D., Harriet Meyer, M.A., Jack Shonkoff, M.D.; and Mickey Segal, Ph.D.

INTRODUCTION

Life has changed for most people living in the United States over the last generation. Families are far more diverse than ever before. Adults have jobs in fields like
Web design and computer programming that did not exist a century ago. Families are
more mobile. Grandparents and grandchildren are often separated by states rather
than neighborhoods. Technology allows families to communicate instantly with writ-
ten words, sounds, and pictures. A volatile economy swings people from prosperity to
poverty in hours. Mothers are more highly educated and more parents are employed.

But what has changed for babies born in the last century? What is the future for
the babies and toddlers of today? There are many stories to tell
about babies and toddlers in the United States. Through the
information in *America's Babies: The ZERO TO THREE Policy
Center Data Book*, we provide a national picture of the well-being
of babies and toddlers, where they live and with whom, and
where they begin the process of lifelong learning. *America's
Babies* offers an overview of some key indicators, available from
data in the public domain, that describe the experiences of
babies and young children during this important phase of their
lives; experiences that will, to a large extent, determine which
pathways of life (or "developmental trajectories") they will follow;
and what their quality of life is and will be in the future. This
information will allow policymakers to better understand how
biological, environmental, and family conditions interact to influence the lifetime development of infants and toddlers.

Many public data sets and compilations of data exist. Some
report child indicators. However, none of these publications
report data specific to infants and toddlers. Most data books
group the child indicators into birth data (e.g., birth rate, birth
weights, etc.), then consolidate the next 5 years. Data that do
exist are often not accessible or interpreted to policymakers in a
way that is meaningful for their work. The lack of data specific
to the first 3 years of life allows this population to be overlooked
in policy discussions.

To remedy this situation, ZERO TO THREE has prepared
this new data book about infants and toddlers. Originally published as *Infants Can't Wait: The Numbers* by ZERO TO THREE
in 1986, this new version provides a similar data-based picture
of the state of infants, toddlers, and families in the United States.
America's Babies includes information drawn primarily from public data sets such as census data and other national data sets.
The data are organized around demographics, child well-being,
family and economic factors, and early educational indicators.
The book is intended to portray the multiple and interrelated
experiences that influence the developmental trajectory of young
children. *America's Babies* provides a visual and graphic repre-
sentation of the key indicators and characteristics of infants, toddlers, and families in the United States as well as newsworthy
changes and trends in the data. Some comparative international

THE CHANGING CIRCUMSTANCES OF BABIES AND TODDLERS

More than 4 decades of knowledge
about early childhood development has
been integrated into a widely acclaimed
report from the National Research Council
and Institute of Medicine. This report, *From
Neurons to Neighborhoods: The Science of
Early Childhood Development* (Shonkoff &
Phillips, 2000), can help inform our thinking
about babies, toddlers, and their families.
From Neurons to Neighborhoods points out
several dramatic transformations in the
social and economic circumstances of
young children and their families. The transformations include the following:

- changes in the nature, schedule, and amount
  of work done by parents of young children;

- struggle to balance work and family
  responsibilities at all income levels;

- economic hardship among families
  despite overall increases in maternal education, increased rates of parent employment, and a strong economy (referring to
  2000 economy);

- increasing cultural diversity;

- significant racial and ethnic disparities in
  health and developmental outcomes;

- growing numbers of babies and young
  children in child care settings of highly
  variable quality; and

- greater awareness of the negative impact
  of serious family problems and community
  conditions on young children.

data (e.g., infant mortality rates, infant morbidity rates, etc.) are included as well. Throughout the book, we use the term *infant* to mean a child under 1 year of age, and *toddler* to mean a child from 1 to 3 years of age.

Babies don't wait. In the first 3 years of life, most babies will learn to smile in response to a smile, cry in response to fear or frustration. Babies will learn to walk, talk, and sing. They will experience the most rapid brain growth of their lives. This amazing growth also creates vulnerability. The brain growth that occurs during the first 3 years is heavily influenced by a baby's experiences and early relationships.

Our hope is that you will find this unique collection of national statistics about the first 3 years of life to be an effective tool in making data-based decisions, and in making sure that America's babies are counted in all that we do.

CINDY OSER AND JULIE COHEN

AMERICA'S BABIES

The ZERO TO THREE Policy Center

DATA BOOK

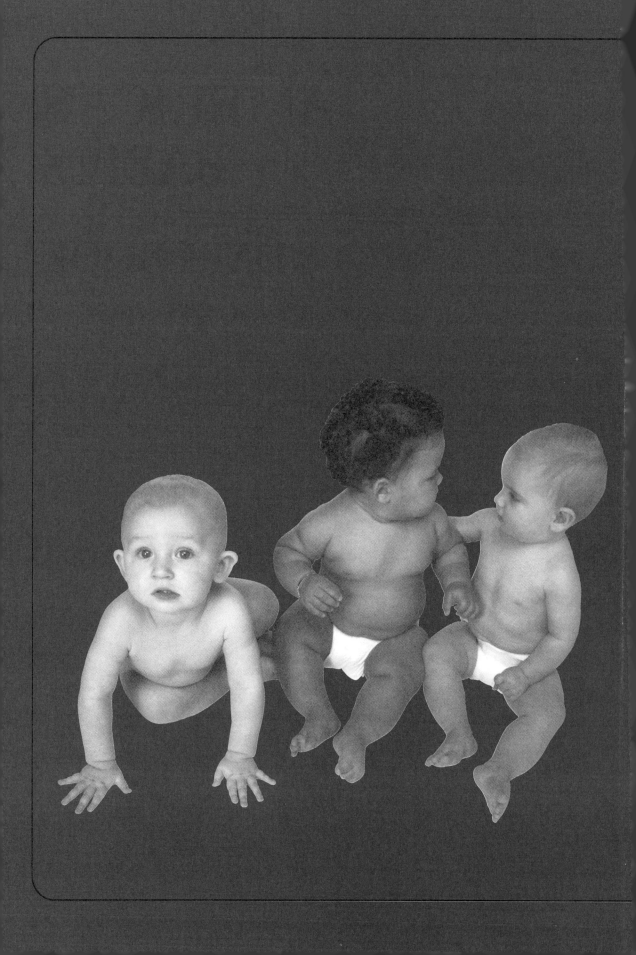

CHAPTER 1
DEMOGRAPHICS OF
BABIES AND TODDLERS

here are 11,416,676 babies and toddlers (birth to age 3) living in the United States (U.S. Census, 2000). This represents 4% of the entire population of the United States. In 2001, there were 4,040,121 babies born (National Center for Health Statistics, 2002a). Approximately 99.3% will survive the first year of life, 51% will survive to age 80, and 1.8% will live to age 100 (Arias, 2002).

The number of children under age 19 in the United States has increased since 1950. This trend is expected to continue over the next 2 decades. Changes in the birth-to-3 population are due to births, deaths, and immigration. This chapter presents basic demographic information about children under age 3 in the United States: how many are born, how many die, what is their race and gender, and where they live.

OVERALL TRENDS

During the "baby boom" (1946 to 1964) the number of children grew rapidly. During the first year of the boom 3.3 million babies arrived — at the time a record number for 1 year. Over 338,000 babies were being born each month, 100,000 more each month than the same month the previous year. From 1954 on, over 4 million babies were born each year, peaking at 4.3 million in 1957. By 1965, the birth rate fell below 4 million; by 1974, the annual birth rate was 3.1 million.

The rising number of annual births between 1977 and 1990 is referred to as the "baby boom echo." The baby boom echo began in the late 1970s and reached 4.1 million births at its peak in 1990, reflecting a 25% increase from 1977. Unlike the decline in the post-baby boom era, when births dropped to 3.1 million in the early 1970s, the number of births in the post-baby boom echo era is expected to remain fairly stable at nearly 4 million for about a decade. Long-range projections by the U.S. Bureau of the Census indicate a rising number of births thereafter, from 4.2 million in 2010 to 4.8 million in 2028, establishing a "millenni-boom" (U.S. Department of Education, 2000).

Figure 1.1 shows the baby boom, the baby boom "echo," and the "millenni-boom" projected for 2010. Trends in live births, births to women ages 15–19 years, and infant mortality are presented in Figures 1.2–1.6.

BIRTHS

There were 4,040,121 babies born in 2001, slightly fewer than in 2000. As the echo baby boomers enter their childbearing years, 4.5 million births (each year) are

> **There are 11,416,676 babies and toddlers (birth to age 3) living in the United States.**
>
> —U.S. Census, 2000

projected by 2020 — exceeding the 4.3 million births recorded in 1957, the height of the baby boom. Still, the annual rate of births is falling (from 16.7 per 1,000 in 1990 to 14.5 per 1,000 in 2001).

Virtually the same number of baby boys and girls are born each year. In 2000, there were 1,048 males born for every 1,000 females (Martin, Hamilton, Ventura, Menacker, & Park, 2002). Although slightly more boys are born than girls, boys are more vulnerable to health conditions such as prematurity, developmental disabilities, accidents, and infant mortality. By the age of 15 years, the ratio of boys to girls approaches 1 to 1. The infant mortality rate is also higher for baby boys (7.6 deaths per 1,000 live births) than for baby girls (6.2 deaths per 1,000 live births).

MYTH: More boys than girls are born each year.

FACT: Virtually the same number of baby boys and girls are born each year.

No industrialized country has a replacement-level birth rate (i.e., the number of births per woman required to replace the population). The overall replacement birth rate is 2.1. Annual total fertility rates for women in the U.S. varied from 4.0 births per woman at the turn of the century, to 3.7 births in 1957, to 1.8 births per woman in the 1980s, to 2.0 in 2001 (Bachu & O'Connell, 2000; (Martin, Park, & Sutton, 2002). This means that based on the birth rate, the overall population of the United States is projected to decrease. Compared to European countries, the United States is growing rapidly because of a higher birth rate and higher immigration (Population Reference Bureau, 2003a).

DEATHS

The infant mortality rate (also called "infant death rate") in the United States has dropped significantly over the last 30 years, from a rate of 20 infant deaths per 1,000 live births in 1970 to 6.9 per 1,000 in 2001. Life expectancy of a newborn has increased to 76.9 years in 2000 (Health Resources Services Administration Maternal and Child Health Bureau, 2002). Infant mortality has decreased over the past 50 years.

Mortality and life expectancy are used as key indicators of overall population

Figure 1.1 Annual Number of Births,
With Projections, 1952–2012

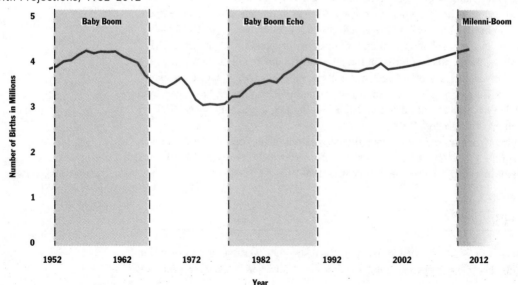

Source: U.S. Department of Education, 2000

health. Some of the change in these indicators has been quite dramatic. For example, between 1950 and 1999 the infant mortality rate nationally declined by 75%. Both neonatal (at the time of birth) and post-neonatal (within the first 28 days of life) infant mortality rates decreased over the last two decades. Mortality rates were highest for babies born to African American women, followed by babies born to American Indian women.

Babies born at very low birth weight — 500 to 999 grams, or a little over 1 pound to about 2 pounds, at birth — now survive at a higher rate than ever before. In 1983, more than half of all babies who weighed 1 pound at birth died before their first birthday. In 2000, babies born weighing 1 pound had a 70% chance of surviving past their first birthday.

IMMIGRATION

The demographics of babies in the United States are changing. There is increasing diversity due to continuing immigration. The current population includes 32.5 million foreign-born residents (11.5% of the population) (Schmidley, 2003).

Between 1970 and 1998, the foreign-born population of the U.S. increased from 9.6 million to 24.4 million. Approximately one third of the U.S. foreign-born population immigrated to the U.S. since 1990. However, the percent of the foreign-born population in the U.S. was lower in 1998 (9%) than in 1900 (14%). Immigration accounts for approximately 30% of the annual population increase in the United States (Population Reference Bureau, 2003a).

Although statistics are not available specific to the

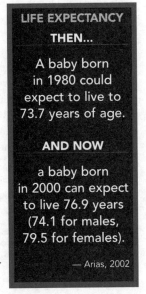

LIFE EXPECTANCY

THEN...

A baby born in 1980 could expect to live to 73.7 years of age.

AND NOW

a baby born in 2000 can expect to live 76.9 years (74.1 for males, 79.5 for females).

— Arias, 2002

Figure 1.2. Annual Live Births
in the United States, 1970–2000

Figure 1.3. Overall Birth Rate Among
Teens Ages 15–19, 1950–2000

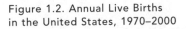

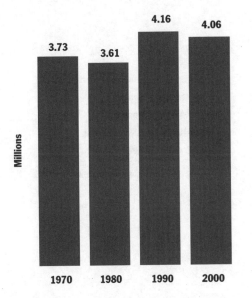

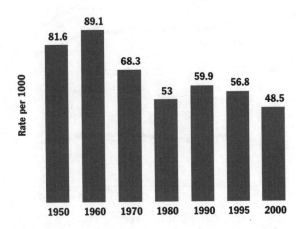

Source: Martin, Hamilton, Ventura, Menacker, & Park, 2002

Source: Martin, Hamilton, Ventura, Menacher, & Park, 2002

birth-to-3 population, 19% of children under age 18 in 2001 lived with at least one parent who was foreign-born[1]; 15% were native and 4% were foreign-born children (Federal Interagency Forum on Child and Family Statistics, 2002). Today, 85% of immigration to the U.S. comes from non-European areas including Asia and South and Central America.

Of all births in the U.S. in 2000, 20% were to Hispanic women, compared with 14% in 1990 (Martin, Hamilton, Ventura, Menacker, & Park, 2002). By 2050, half of all Americans will be non-white. Hispanics and Asians will account for 61% of population growth in the U.S. over the next 20 years (44% Hispanic, 17% Asian).

Educational levels differ for native and foreign-born parents. "The percentage of children whose parents have less than a high school diploma is much higher among children with at least one foreign-born parent than among children with native parents" (Federal Interagency Forum on Child and Family Statistics, 2002, p. 58). In 2001, 42% of foreign-born children with at least one foreign-born parent had less than a high school degree; 35% of native children with at least one foreign-born parent, and 11% of native children with native parents, had less than a high school degree.

Foreign-born children with foreign-born parents were more likely than native children with foreign-born parents to live in poverty.

The population of the U.S. represents a variety of races and ethnicities. Child bearing and child rearing are influenced by cultural traditions. Some aspects of child well-being, such as the low birth weight rate, seem to be associated with race but may also be influenced by other factors such as access to health care, poverty, and smoking during pregnancy.

The 2000 Census allowed people to mark more than one race, allowing for the first time a national count of the multi-racial population in the U.S. Of the 281.4 mil-

By 2050, half of all Americans will be non-white.

---

[1] Foreign-born means the individual was not a U.S. citizen at birth. Native means the individual was born in the United States or a U.S. Island Area such as Puerto Rico or was born abroad of a U.S. citizen parent (Schmidley, 2003).

Figure 1.4. Births to Teens Ages 15–19 by Race, 1980–2000

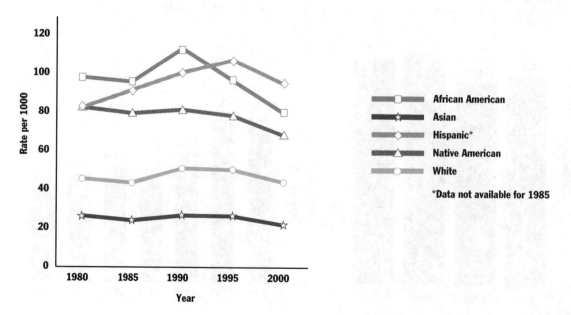

Legend:
- African American
- Asian
- Hispanic*
- Native American
- White

*Data not available for 1985

Source: Martin, Hamilton, Ventura, Menacker, & Park, 2002

lion people counted in the 2000 Census, 6.8 million (2.4%) identified themselves as multi-racial. The most common bi-racial mix was white and American Indian/Alaska Native (1 million), followed by white and Asian (868,000), white and black (785,000), and black and American Indian/Alaska native (182,000). The multi-racial population

Figure 1.5. Infant Mortality Rates by Mother's Race, 1983–2000

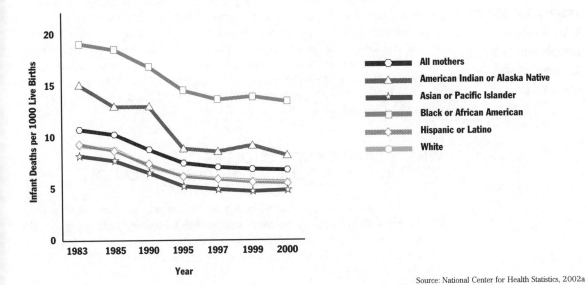

Source: National Center for Health Statistics, 2002a

Figure 1.6. Infant Mortality Rates by Birth Weight, 1983–2000.

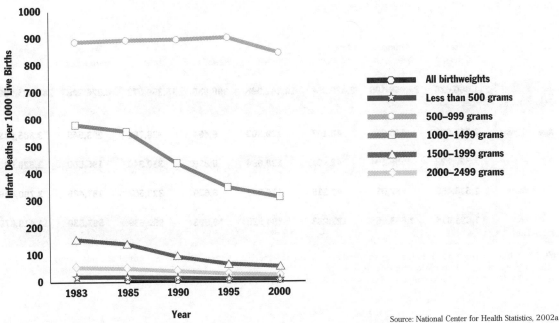

Source: National Center for Health Statistics, 2002a

also included 3.2 million people who identified themselves as Hispanic/Latino. More children were identified as multi-racial (4%) as compared with adults (2%) (Jones & Smith, 2001; Mather, 2000).

Services and service providers, including those in schools, child care, hospitals, and health care, are called upon to respond to increasing diversity in the languages and traditions of families in the United States. At least 40% of all Americans have had some racial mixing in the last three generations, but only 2 to 4% will indicate this on Census 2000. The blurring of racial categories will blur even faster as children of Asian and Hispanic immigrants are marrying out of their parents' heritage at rates between 30% and 60%. Today, only 15% of European Americans are married to a spouse from the same country of origin (Hodgkinson, 2001).

In 2000, there were approximately equal numbers of children – between 23 and 24 million – in each age group: birth to 5, 6 to 11, and 12 to 17 years of age. The number of infants and toddlers was also distributed nearly equally across ages birth to 1 (3,805,648), 1 to 2 (3,820,582) and 2 to 3 (3,790,446; Federal Interagency Forum on Child and Family Statistics, 2002). It is estimated that the birth-to-3 population will increase slightly over the next 20 years.

> **Most migration occurs within states, but about 6 to 8 million people move to another state each year.**
>
> —Hodgkinson, 2001

WHERE BABIES AND TODDLERS LIVE: DISTRIBUTION OF THE BIRTH-TO-3 POPULATION

Up to 40 million Americans move each year. Most migration occurs within states, but about 6 to 8 million people move to another state each year (Hodgkinson, 2001).

More than half of the population of the United States resides in only nine states (California, Florida, Illinois, Michigan, New Jersey, New York, Ohio, Pennsylvania, and Texas). As the diversity of our population increases, the increase in diversity will be absorbed by about 230 of the 3,068 counties in the United States, and three states (California, Texas, and Florida) will absorb about 60% of the increasing diversity (Hodgkinson, 2001).

Table 1.1. Birth-to-3 Population by Race, 2000

	White American	African-American	American-Indian	Asian	Hawaiian	Other	Two or more races	Total all races
Total U.S. Population	211,460,626	34,658,190	2,475,956	10,242,998	398,835	15,359,073	6,826,228	281,421,906
Age < 1 year	2,535,928	548,955	42,167	129,803	6,464	338,786	203,545	3,805,648
1 – 2 years	2,557,128	556,194	42,901	130,694	6,819	330,346	196,500	3,820,582
2 – 3 years	2,538,459	557,919	42,215	134,241	6,620	323,507	187,485	3,790,446
Total birth to 3 years	7,631,515	1,663,068	127,283	394,738	19,903	992,639	587,530	11,416,676

NOTE: Table 1.1 does not break out Hispanic/Latino because the U.S. Census Bureau defines Hispanic/Latino as an ethnicity, not a race. Population figures for this group in 2000 were: Age < 1year—771,053; 1–2 years—745,686; 2–3 years—731,495; and total birth to 3 years—2,248,234.

Source: http://factfinder.census.gov

Table 1.2. Birth-to-3 Population by State, 2000

	% of whole population	Age < 1 year	Age 1–2 years	Age 2–3	Total 0–3
Total United States (excludes Puerto Rico)	5.42%	3,805,648	3,820,582	3,790,446	11,416,676
Alabama	5.31%	59,101	59,123	58,875	177,099
Alaska	6.02%	9,361	9,467	9,403	28,231
Arizona	5.96%	77,421	77,174	75,241	229,836
Arkansas	5.42%	36,065	36,258	36,232	108,555
California	5.80%	483,143	486,587	489,336	1,459,066
Colorado	5.53%	60,823	60,036	58,271	179,130
Connecticut	5.19%	42,719	44,435	43,659	130,813
Delaware	5.22%	10,286	10,347	10,234	30,867
District of Columbia	4.50%	6,518	6,280	6,478	19,276
Florida	4.70%	186,977	187,793	187,069	561,839
Georgia	5.81%	120,992	120,003	117,260	358,255
Hawaii	5.11%	15,464	15,571	15,377	46,412
Idaho	6.03%	19,700	19,745	19,105	58,550
Illinois	5.60%	173,373	174,005	173,172	520,550
Indiana	5.54%	84,517	84,828	83,791	253,136
Iowa	5.13%	37,338	37,786	37,364	112,488
Kansas	5.60%	37,977	38,235	37,244	113,456
Kentucky	5.25%	53,156	53,682	52,681	159,519
Louisiana	5.68%	64,092	63,992	63,202	191,286
Maine	4.38%	13,456	14,013	13,984	41,453
Maryland	5.29%	69,647	70,265	69,306	209,218
Massachuetts	4.97%	77,998	78,949	79,011	235,958
Michigan	5.37%	131,188	133,680	133,732	398,600
Minnesota	5.33%	65,072	65,749	65,168	195,989
Mississippi	5.73%	41,217	41,192	40,669	123,078
Missouri	5.26%	72,842	74,277	73,949	221,068
Montana	4.83%	10,732	11,002	10,798	32,532
Nebraska	5.46%	23,459	23,684	22,963	70,106
Nevada	5.81%	29,046	29,163	28,558	86,767
New Hampshire	4.82%	14,006	14,839	15,052	43,897
New Jersey	5.31%	110,298	111,308	111,529	333,135
New Mexico	5.72%	26,335	26,381	25,622	78,338
New York	5.17%	243,891	244,103	244,071	732,065
North Carolina	5.37%	110,654	109,289	106,592	326,535
North Dakota	4.87%	7,660	7,754	7,943	23,357
Ohio	5.28%	148,468	150,266	149,956	448,690
Oklahoma	5.50%	47,533	48,123	47,521	143,177
Oregon	5.19%	44,189	44,355	44,190	132,734
Pennsylvania	4.68%	141,431	143,368	143,475	428,274
Rhode Island	4.83%	12,206	12,778	12,791	37,775
South Carolina	5.27%	53,947	52,971	52,469	159,387
South Dakota	5.40%	10,239	10,357	9,920	30,516
Tennessee	5.25%	75,127	75,444	74,254	224,825
Texas	6.23%	330,770	325,393	321,275	977,438
Utah	7.60%	44,605	43,368	41,227	129,200
Vermont	4.40%	6,381	6,767	6,659	19,807
Virginia	5.21%	92,708	92,746	91,160	276,614
Washington	5.33%	77,740	78,919	78,816	235,475
West Virginia	4.47%	20,176	20,145	20,083	60,404
Wisconsin	5.07%	67,474	68,283	67,582	203,339
Wyoming	5.01%	6,130	6,304	6,127	18,561
Puerto Rico	6.15%	58,043	57,673	59,133	174,849

Source: U.S. Census, 2000

Figure 1.7. Birth-to-3 Population 1950–2000 and Projected 2001–2020

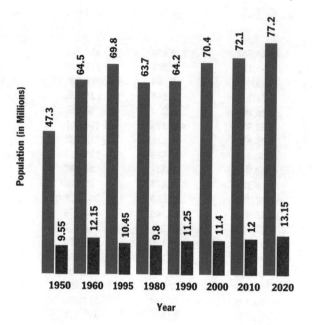

Total U.S. population under age 18

Total U.S. population age birth to 3

NOTE: All population figures for the year 2000 shown here are estimates based on the 1990 Census; They do not reflect Census 2000 counts. Population figures for 2001–2020 are projections.

Source: U.S. Census Bureau, Population Estimates and Projections, 2002.

Figure 1.8. U.S. 2000 Census Average Percent Population Birth-to-3 by State

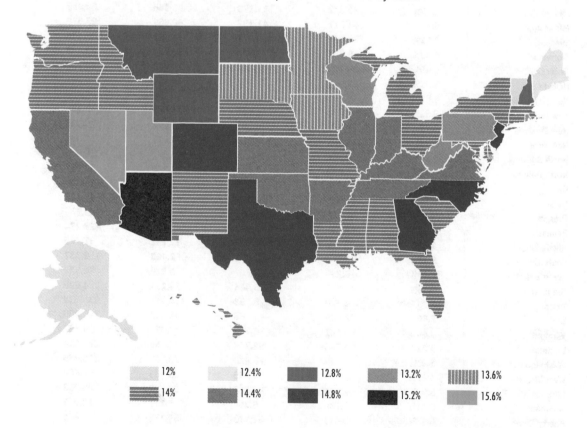

12%   12.4%   12.8%   13.2%   13.6%
14%   14.4%   14.8%   15.2%   15.6%

Source: U.S. Census, 2000

Figure 1.9. U.S. 2000 Census Average Population Birth-to-3 by State

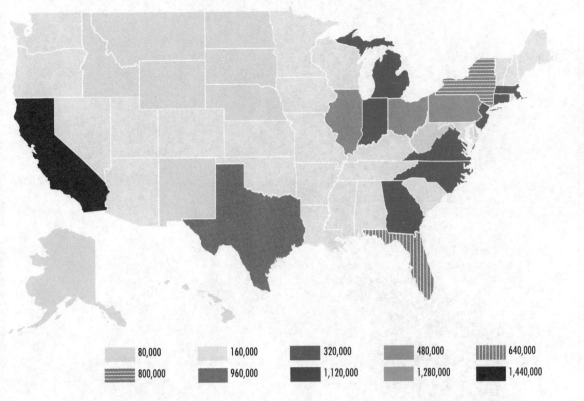

80,000		160,000		320,000		480,000		640,000
800,000		960,000		1,120,000		1,280,000		1,440,000

Source: U.S. Census, 2000

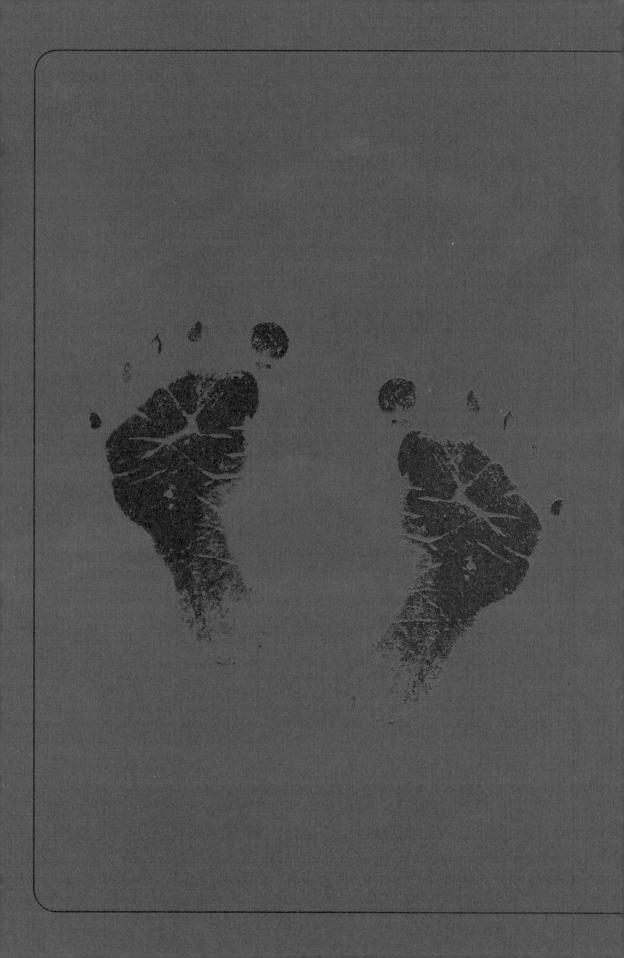

CHAPTER 2
BABIES, COMING INTO THE WORLD

growing body of evidence calls attention to the tremendous opportunity for improving the potential for optimal development that exists during a child's first years of life. Eighty-five percent of brain growth occurs in the first 3 years of life. During this time, the brain is growing neurons and synapses, making connections and "wiring" for important aspects of brain development, including those important in cognition, perception, behavior, and communication. In addition to physical brain growth, the foundation for the health and development of each child is being built during these few years. Babies and toddlers develop competencies in the context of close personal relationships and in their day-to-day interactions with the important people in their lives. What each child experiences during this period of rapid physical and mental growth — both positive and negative — will influence how and what he or she learns (Shonkoff & Phillips, 2000). These developments are, in turn, critical for expansion of social and learning skills that are needed to function appropriately later in life. Recent evidence suggests that even basic adaptive physiological response systems, measured in adulthood, have been influenced by environmental events that occurred during the prenatal or early childhood experience. These findings underscore the importance of understanding how early life experiences can be used to promote optimal lifetime health and well-being.

In 2000, there were 2,839,000 babies and toddlers living in poverty in the U.S.

— U.S. Bureau of Labor Statistics, 2001b.

In this chapter, a number of key indicators of child well-being are identified. Although not all indicators are reported in a form that permits explicit identification of children under age 3, some general trends in measures of child health, economic security, and social/environmental living conditions are presented.

Overall, the data suggest a correlation between economic status and health status for children in general. Based on data from the National Health Interview Survey for 2000 (National Center for Health Statistics, 2002b), a smaller percentage of children (70%) living in households with incomes below the poverty line were reported to be in very good or excellent health as compared with those in households with incomes at or above the poverty line (85%). This effect has been evident since at least 1984. The general trend over this same time period reflects a gradual improvement in health status and a small decrease in the extent of the disparity.

Very low birth weight rates (babies born at or below 1,500 grams, or about 3.3 pounds), in particular, continue to show disparity between African American and other populations.

The relationship between economic conditions and health may be mediated by maternal education level and other factors such as early educational experiences. These will be explored in Chapters 3 and 6.

WHERE AND HOW BABIES ARE BORN

Of all babies born in the United States in 2000, 88% are delivered in hospitals by physicians (medical doctors and osteopathic physicians, see Table 2.1). There has been an increase in the number of deliveries by certified nurse midwives, from 4% in 1990 to 7% in 2000.

EARLY HOSPITAL DISCHARGE: WHATEVER HAPPENED TO "DRIVE-THROUGH DELIVERIES?"

In 1970, the average length of stay for all hospital deliveries was 4.1 days (median: 4 days). By 1992, the average had decreased to 2.6 days (median: 2.0 days). The average length of stay for women who gave birth vaginally decreased by 46% (from 3.9 to 2.1 days) and for those who gave birth by cesarean section by 49% (from 7.8 to 4.0 days, see Tables 2.2 and 2.3). In 1997, the average length of stay following delivery was 2.4 days (Centers for Disease Control and Prevention, 1995, 2002a).

In the mid-1990s, some insurance companies and hospitals were requiring mothers and babies to be discharged 24 hours following delivery. In response to concern that early postpartum discharge might lead to serious complications in mothers and babies, the U.S. Congress passed legislation in 1996 requiring that women be allowed to stay in the hospital for 48 hours after childbirth (72 hours after a C-section); the law went into effect in 1998. Studies conducted after implementation of this law concluded that early postpartum discharge policies do not seem to affect health outcomes of newborn babies, and the policies had minimal effect on hospital expenditures (Madden et al., 2002).

Table 2.1. Location of Births, 1990–2000

	1990	1995	2000
Total Births	4,162,917	3,903,012	4,058,814
Hospital	4,112,481	3,862,605	4,020,877
Freestanding birthing center	16,063	11,749	10,738
Clinic or doctor's office	1,133	882	466
Residence	27,967	24,397	23,843
Other	3,633	2,656	2,588
Unknown or not stated	1,640	723	302

Source: Martin, Hamilton, Ventura, Menacker, & Park, 2002

Table 2.2. Methods of Delivery, 2000

Vaginal deliveries	3,108,888
Cesarean deliveries (primary)	577,638
Cesarean deliveries (repeat)	346,353
Cesarean delivery rate	22.9%

Source: Martin, Hamilton, Ventura, Menacker, & Park, 2002

ASSISTIVE REPRODUCTIVE TECHNOLOGY

The first U.S-born baby conceived through in-vitro fertilization was delivered in 1981, 3 years after the first-ever baby conceived by in-vitro fertilization was born in England (American Society for Reproductive Medicine, 2003b). In-vitro fertilization, one type of assisted reproductive technology, is a medical response to infertility. Infertility is a condition of the reproductive system that impairs the body's ability to perform the basic functions of reproduction (American Society for Reproductive Medicine, 2003c). Infertility affects about 6.1 million people in the U.S. — about 10% of the reproductive age population. Infertility affects men and women equally. Most infertility — 85% to 90% — is treated with conventional medical therapies such as medication or surgery. For less than 5% of patients with infertility, assistive reproductive technologies (ART) such as in-vitro fertilization are used.

The number of babies conceived through ART is on the rise. In 1998, 20,143 live births resulted from ART procedures (Schieve, Jeng, Wilcox & Reynolds, 2002). In 2000, there were 35,025 live births resulted from ART; this represents fewer than 1% of all births. Of these births, 35% (12,258 babies) were multiples (twins or higher), compared to a multiple birth rate of 3% in the general population. The incidence of birth defects in children resulting from in vitro fertilization is the same as the incidence in children conceived naturally (American Society for Reproductive Medicine, 2003b).

In 2002, 3% of the babies born through ART (1,050 babies) were triplets or higher-order births, down from 5% in 1999 (American Society for Reproductive Medicine, 1999). In response to concerns about increasing rates of high-order multiple births, new guidelines were released in January 2000, recommending the number of embryos or eggs to be transferred (American Society for Reproductive Medicine, 1999). The average cost of one in-vitro fertilization cycle is $8,000–$10,000.

The rate of triplets and higher-order multiple births has increased 400% in the past two decades.

—Martin, Hamilton, Ventura, Menacker, Park & Sutton, 2002

Table 2.3. Births by Delivery Attendant

	1990	1995	2000
Total attended births	4,162,917	3,903,012	4,058,814
Doctor of medicine (M.D.)	3,824,822	3,498,586	3,553,187
Doctor of osteopathy (D.O.)	126,679	142,062	168,644
Certified nurse midwife (C.N.M.)	148,781	218,710	297,902
Other midwife	15,682	14,597	16,637
Other	30,760	22,206	21,325
Unknown or not stated	16,193	6,851	1,119

Source: Martin, Hamilton, Ventura, Menacker, & Park, 2002

MULTIPLE BIRTHS

The percentage of babies born prematurely in the United States reached a 20-year high in 2001, driven by an increase in twins and triplets (see Table 2.4). The increase in multiples is due in part to the increase in assistive reproductive technology, including in vitro fertilization. Only 1.2% of natural pregnancies result in twins while 40% of women under age 35 who become pregnant through in-vitro fertilization will deliver twins. The increase in multiple births is also attributed to the older age of childbearing. Health care costs for delivery and newborn care is four times higher than for a singleton birth. The costs are 12 times higher for triplets (American Society for Reproductive Medicine, 2003a).

Multiple birth pregnancies are risky for the babies and for the mothers. These pregnancies have higher rates of caesarean section, prematurity, low birth weight, and infant death and disability. Normal pregnancies last 37–42 weeks. Twins are born, on average, at 35 weeks, triplets at 33 weeks, and quadruplets at 30 weeks. Most of these babies will be healthy, but many of these multiples will be born extremely prematurely — at 28 weeks or less — when babies are most vulnerable to lung problems, infection, bleeding in the brain, and other disabilities.

BIRTH WEIGHT

The average full-term baby in the United States weighs 7 pounds (3,275 grams) at birth (Beers & Berkow, 1999). Birth weight is one indicator of health at birth. Low birth weight (less than 5 pounds 8 ounces, or 2,500 grams) and very low birth weight (less than 3 pounds 4 ounces or 1,500 grams) are associated with higher rates of infant mortality, learning disabilities, and physical and mental disabilities (see Table 2.5, Figure 2.1, and Figure 2.2).

Table 2.4. Multiple Births, 2000

Annual multiple births	128,717
Twin births	121,246
Triplet births	6,885
Quadruplet births	501
Quintuplet and higher	85

Table 2.5. Birth Weight Data, 2000

Median weight at birth	6.6–7.7 pounds (3,000–3,499 grams)
Annual number of preterm births	467,201 (11.6%)
Annual number of babies born low birthweight	307,030 (7.6%)
Annual number of babies with very low birth weight	56,826 (1.4%)

Source: Martin, Hamilton, Ventura, Menacker, & Park, 2002.

Source: Martin, Hamilton, Ventura, Menacker, & Park, 2002.

FACTORS AFFECTING BIRTH SIZE AND BIRTH OUTCOME: SMOKING AND DRUG USE DURING PREGNANCY

Smoking during pregnancy is known to be a risk factor for low birth weight and infant mortality. In 1990, 18.4% of pregnant women smoked cigarettes during pregnancy; 12% of pregnant women smoked cigarettes in 2000 (Mathews, 2001). In the general population, 21% of all women are cigarette smokers (National Center for Health Statistics, 2002a). Mothers age 18–19 are still more likely to smoke than mothers in other age groups, but a decrease in the smoking rate in this subgroup was seen in 2000, reversing the increase trend observed over the 5 previous years. The effects of smoking and birth weight are shown in Figures 2.3 and 2.4.

Alcohol use during pregnancy causes mental retardation and other disabilities. This set of developmental characteristics, usually evident at birth, is known as Fetal Alcohol Syndrome. Alcohol use during pregnancy does not always result in Fetal Alcohol Syndrome. Individuals may be affected by prenatal alcohol exposure but may not have the characteristic facial abnormalities and growth retardation associated with Fetal Alcohol Syndrome. Two terms are used to describe this type of affect: Alcohol-Related Neurodevelopmental Disorder (ARND), a condition where there are functional or mental impairments linked to prenatal alcohol exposure, and Alcohol-Related Birth Defects (ARBD), a condition where the individual has abnormalities in the skeletal and major organ systems due to prenatal alcohol exposure (National Organization on Fetal Alcohol Syndrome, 2003).

At least 12,000 infants are born each year with Fetal Alcohol Syndrome, and three times as many with ARND or ARBD. The 2001 National Household Survey on Drug Abuse (NHSDA) reports an alcohol use rate of 12.9% among pregnant women (compared to 49.8% of non-pregnant women and 2.4% of women with children less than 1 year of age; National Household Survey on Drug Abuse, 2001). Many women reduce or curtail their use of alcohol and cigarettes during pregnancy. NHSDA also reported a binge drinking rate (drinking five or more drinks on the same occasion at

Hospital charges for preterm/low birth weight newborns average $51,800 compared with $3,700 for normal newborns

—March of Dimes, 2001

Figure 2.1. Low Birth Weight Births by Race, 1970–2000.

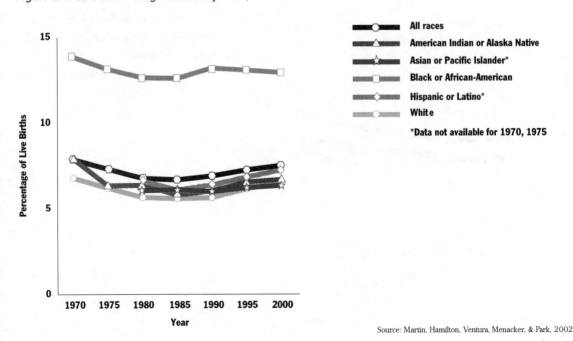

Source: Martin, Hamilton, Ventura, Menacker, & Park, 2002

least once in the past 30 days) of 4.6% among pregnant women age 15 to 44 years. The rate of binge drinking among non-pregnant women is 20.5%. Reductions in tobacco and alcohol use in women during pregnancy are not permanent. Interviews with women who had given birth in the past year indicated that cigarette smoking and binge drinking rates were similar to overall rates for non-pregnant women.

BIRTH DEFECTS

Approximately 3% of all babies born each year will have birth defects or conditions that are present at birth and affect growth and development. Some of these conditions, such as cleft lip/palate or club foot, are correctable. Others, such as Down syndrome or microcephaly, may cause mild to severe mental retardation. These children require longer-term therapies and special education. Selected birth anomalies are shown in Table 2.6.

Figure 2.2. Very Low Birth Weight Births (<1,500 Grams or 3.3 Pounds) by Race, 1980–2000

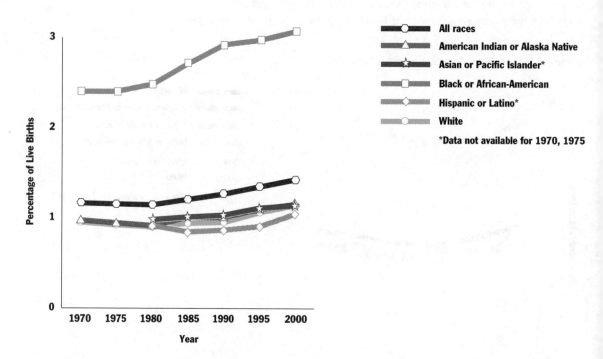

Source: Martin, Hamilton, Ventura, Menacker, & Park, 2002

Figure 2.3. Low Birth Weight (<2,500 Grams or 5 Pounds) by Smoking Status of Mother, 1989–2000

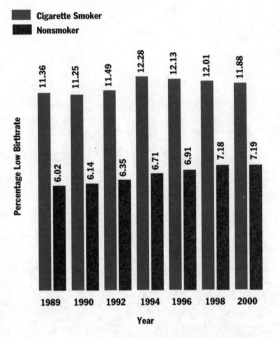

Source: National Center for Health Statistics (2002a)

Figure 2.4. Very Low Birth Weight (<1,500 Grams or 3.3 Pounds) Rates by Smoking Status of Mother, 1989–2000

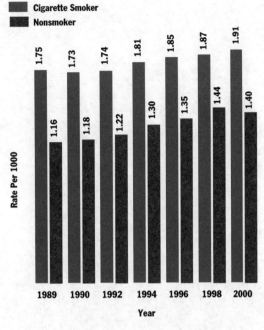

Source: National Center for Health Statistics (2002a)

Table 2.6. Birth Defects Rate per 100,000 Live Births, 1990 and 1999

	1990	1999		1990	1999
Other musculoskeletal/integumental	185	234	Other gastrointestinal	32	29
Other circulatory/respiratory	120	137	Hydrocephalus	26	21
Heart malformation	113	117	Spina bifida/meningocele	23	20
Other urogenital	116	97	Other central nervous system	23	19
Polydactyly/syndactyly/adactyly	79	86	Diaphragmatic hernia	15	13
Cleft lip/palate	77	79	Renal agenesis	8	13
Malformed genitalia	71	74	Tracheo-esophageal fistula/atresia	14	13
Club foot	63	54	Anencephalus	15	11
Down syndrome	48	44	Rectal atresia/stenosis	9	9
Other chromosomal	39	36	Microcephalus	9	6
Omphalocele/gastroschisis	21	29	Other	601	420

Source: Centers for Disease Control and Prevention (2003a)

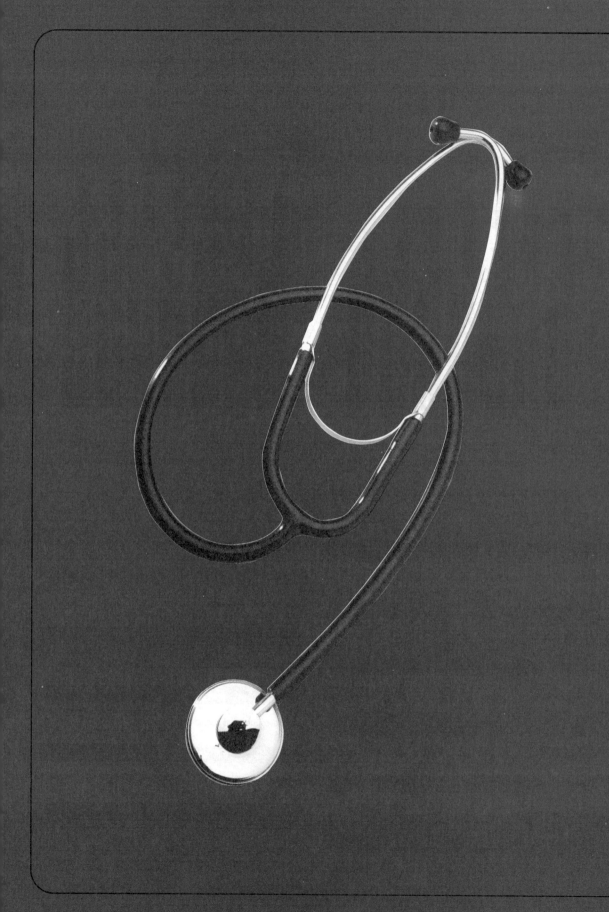

CHAPTER 3
INFANTS AND TODDLERS, HEALTHY AND SAFE

P renatal care and attention to labor, delivery, and the birthing process help to assure better birth outcomes. Beginning immediately after birth, babies encounter a new world and new influences on their health and development. This chapter presents information about some of the preventive measures and environmental exposures that may affect health and development.

It is possible to screen babies for many health conditions at birth. With relatively inexpensive testing, conditions such as deafness, hypothyroidism, sickle cell anemia, and other disorders can be detected and treated before they permanently affect learning, development, and survival. Newborn screening for conditions that are identifiable and treatable at birth is one of the most affordable and prudent ways to promote child well-being.

Each year, 12,000 babies are born with permanent hearing loss.

—National Center for Hearing Assessment and Management, 2003

NEWBORN METABOLIC SCREENING

Nearly every baby born in the United States is screened for a variety of genetic, metabolic, and endocrine disorders immediately after birth. In all states, this screening is mandated by law (except when parents refuse on religious or other grounds). With a few drops of blood obtained by pricking a baby's heel, up to 55 diseases can be screened. All states screen for PKU (phenylketonuria) and congenital hypothyroidism. If untreated, both of these conditions result in mental retardation. Most states also screen for galactosemia and sickle cell disease. Lack of treatment for these conditions can be fatal. Average cost of newborn metabolic screening is $18; in most states, the screening and the follow-up treatment are covered by private insurance, Medicaid, and State Children's Health Insurance Program (March of Dimes and PriceWaterhouseCoopers, 2002).

NEWBORN HEARING SCREENING

Each year, 12,000 babies are born with permanent hearing loss (National Center for Hearing Assessment and Management, 2003). Congenital hearing loss occurs at a rate of 3 in every 1,000 births (Centers for Disease Control and Prevention, 2002c). Children with deafness or hearing impairment are able to develop language, social, and communication skills if the hearing loss is detected early and appropriate intervention is provided. To address this issue, a movement has been underway since the early 1990s to mandate hearing screening for all newborns. As of 2002, 69% of all babies born in the United States are screened for hearing impairment (National

Center for Hearing Assessment and Management, 2003), and 32 states have passed legislation requiring newborn hearing screening.

HEALTH AND NUTRITION

Although much of the brain's structure is established at birth, food provides the nutrients required to fuel the brain's subsequent development and the body's functioning. Babies are fortunate to have most of their nutritional requirements met through breast milk or infant formula. For toddlers, food provides nutrients and calories but also provides an important routine opportunity to interact with caregivers, to try new tastes and textures, and begin to exercise choice and preference. Just as early experiences and relationships lay the foundation for later learning, early nutrition can form healthy (or unhealthy) eating habits and physical health patterns for life.

Nationally, being overweight is a more common problem than being underweight among infants and toddlers. The prevalence of underweight (low weight for height) was 3.1% among children birth to age 2, and 1.9% among children age 2 to 5 years. A national study concluded that severe malnutrition did not seem to be a significant public health problem for young children who participated in the study (Centers for Disease Control and Prevention, 1998b).

Overweight is on the rise, even among infants and toddlers. Among children birth to age 2, the prevalence of overweight was 10.8% in 1989, rising to 11.3% in 1997. Among children age 2 to 5, prevalence rose from 7.0% in 1987 to 8.6% in 1997.

Obesity (weight that is 120% of ideal body weight or a body mass index [BMI] greater than 85% for age) is also a growing problem for children in the United States. It is the most common nutritional disorder in children; as many as 1 in 4 children is obese. In adults, obesity is an important risk factor for cardiovascular disease (Barlow & Dietz, 1998; von Kries et al., 1999). Infant weight appears to correlate strongly with adult weight independently of other factors such as social class, educational level,

Table 3.1. Then and Now: Breast-feeding, 1974–2000

1974:	30% of all babies breast-fed in hospital after birth
1994:	58% of all babies breast-fed in hospital after birth
2000:	68% of all babies breast-fed in hospital after birth
1974:	62.3% of all babies breast-fed for 3 months or more
1994:	56.2% of all babies breast-fed for 3 months or more
2000:	31% of all babies still breast-fed at 6 months of age

Figure 3.1. Breast-feeding by Race, 2000

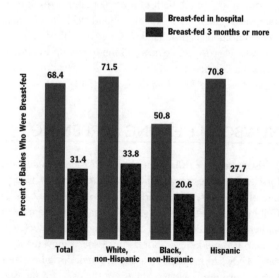

Source: National Center for Health Statistics, 2002a; Health Resources Services Administration, Maternal and Child Health Bureau, 2002

Source: Martin, Hamilton, Ventura, Menacher, & Park, 2002

and parental weight (Charney, Goodman, McBride, Lyon, & Pratt, 1976; Phillips & Young, 2000).

Prolonged breast-feeding may help decrease the prevalence of obesity in childhood (von Kries et al., 1999). A national study concluded that among infants who were not exclusively breast-fed, those who were fed more breast-milk than infant formula, or who were breast-fed for longer periods, had a lower risk of being overweight during later childhood and adolescence (Gillman, 2001).

BREAST-FEEDING

Breast milk is the preferred nutrition for human babies. It contains antibodies that protect newborns from infections until their own immune systems mature. It is recommended that babies be exclusively breast-fed for the first 6 months of life (American Academy of Pediatrics, 1997). The national health objective for breast-feeding is that 75% of all babies are breast-fed early (starting right after birth, in the hospital) and 50% will continue to be breast-fed exclusively until 6 months of age (U.S. Department of Health and Human Services, 2000a). These goals have not been met (see Table 3.1). Data from the 2001 Ross Laboratories Mothers Survey (RLMS) indicate that national breast-feeding rates have reached an all-time high, with 69.5% of mothers breast-feeding in the hospital immediately after birth, and 32.5% of babies who continue to be fed breast milk at 6 months of age (Ryan, Wenjun, & Acosta, 2002). Figure 3.1 displays current breast-feeding rates by race/ethnicity.

Breast-feeding is more beneficial than formula feeding for infants. Infants who are breast-fed have resistance to bacterial and viral infectious diseases such as diarrhea, respiratory tract infections, otitis media (ear infections), and pneumonia. Breast-fed infants have enhanced immune systems and have fewer illnesses than infants who were never breast-fed.

Mothers benefit from breast-feeding, too. Mothers who breast-fed their babies experience less postpartum bleeding, an earlier return to pre-pregnancy weight, and a reduced risk of ovarian cancer and pre-menopausal cancer. A recent meta-analysis of 47 studies conducted in 30 countries and including more than 50,000 women concluded that the number of children women have and the length of time they breast-feed them are important factors influencing their chance of developing breast cancer. The researchers estimated that if women in developed countries delayed weaning by 6 months, they could reduce breast cancer risk by 5% — perhaps 25,000 fewer cases of cancer per year (Beral et al., 2002).

Breast milk is less expensive than commercial infant formula.

Breast milk = $0.96/quart (additional food eaten by the mother)

Infant formula = $1.90/quart

—University Medical Center Tucson Arizona, 2003

THE WOMEN, INFANTS, AND CHILDREN (WIC) SUPPLEMENTAL NUTRITION PROGRAM

The Special Supplemental Nutrition Program for Women, Infants, and Children (WIC), established as a pilot program in 1972 and made permanent in 1974, was created to help alleviate the effects of poverty on the health of infants, children, and pregnant or new mothers. Benefits provided to WIC participants are: supplemental nutritious foods; nutrition education and counseling at WIC clinics; and screening and referrals to other health, welfare, and social services. To receive WIC services, participants must be eligible by income (185% of the federal poverty level), nutritional risk, and category (either a pregnant, breast-feeding, or postpartum woman; an infant under 1 year old; or a child under 5 years old).

WIC is not considered an entitlement program; Congress does not set aside funds to allow every qualified individual to participate in the program. WIC is a federal grant program for which Congress authorizes a specific amount of funds each year. The program is administered by the Food and Nutrition Service of the U.S. Department of Agriculture. WIC serves about 81% of all eligible women, infants, and children (U.S. Department of Agriculture Food and Nutrition Service, 2002). Tables 3.2 and 3.3 display current enrollment data.

Infant Formula Sales:

27–28 billion ounces of infant formula are sold each year.

In 2000, sales reached $2.9 billion dollars

—U.S. Department of Agriculture Economic Research Service, 2001

PHYSICAL ACTIVITY FOR BABIES

"Confining babies and young children to strollers, play pens, [or] car and infant seats for hours at a time, may delay development such as rolling over, crawling, walking and even cognitive development" (National Association for Sport and Physical Education, 2002). Lack of prone positioning (with babies on their stomach) during non-sleep time is associated with an increase in a condition called torticollis (neck muscles that are stronger on one side than the other, leading to lopsided muscle strength and a preference for keeping the head turned to one side), plagiocephaly (flattened head), and gross motor delay (Raco, Raimondi, DePonte, & Brunelli, 1999; Kane, Mitchell, Craven, & Marsh, 1996).

As a companion to the "Back to Sleep" campaign, "Tummy Time to Play" is promoted to encourage babies to explore their environment, strengthen muscles needed for head control, and for future crawling, standing, and walking (Pontius et al., 2001). Prone sleeping (on the back) does not seem to affect long-term motor development. Although infants who sleep on their backs do not crawl as early as babies who sleep on their stomachs, they soon become just as mobile (Davis, Moon, Sachs & Ottolini, 1998).

Infants should be encouraged to interact with parents and/or caregivers during physical activities, be physically active, and to explore their environments from the

Table 3.2. Then and Now: WIC Participation

Year	Participation
1974	88,000
1980	1.9 million
1990	4.5 million
2000	7.2 million

Table 3.3. Average Monthly WIC Participation, 2001

Of the 7.31 million women, infants, and children served each month:

1.92 million are infants under age 1

3.61 million are children under age 5

1.78 million are pregnant or postpartum women

Source: U.S. Department of Agriculture Food and Nutrition Service, 2002   Source: U.S. Department of Agriculture Food and Nutrition Service, 2002

beginning of life. Physical activity guidelines specifically designed to meet the developmental needs of infants, toddlers, and preschoolers were issued for the first time in 2001 (National Association for Sport and Physical Education, 2002).

PUBLIC PREVENTIVE HEALTH: THE EARLY AND PERIODIC SCREENING, DIAGNOSIS, AND TREATMENT (EPSDT) PROGRAM

The Early and Periodic Screening, Diagnosis, and Treatment (EPSDT) program is Medicaid's comprehensive and preventive child health program. EPSDT has been part of the federal Medicaid program since the late 1960s. EPSDT provisions entitle children who meet financial eligibility to a comprehensive package of preventive health care and medically necessary diagnosis and treatment and includes periodic screening, vision, dental, and hearing services for children under the age of 21. Congress increased the services of EPSDT through the Omnibus Budget Reconciliation Act of 1989. States must now cover regular and periodic screenings for all eligible children. They must also provide any medically necessary services indicated by the screenings, even those not covered in a state's Medicaid plan.

The health screenings provided under EPSDT are intended to identify and correct any treatable problems early in the child's life to prevent further deterioration. Nearly 80% of all eligible infants are participating in EPSDT. Approximately 55% of children ago 1–5 are participating. Twenty percent of all children age 1–5 are receiving dental screenings. Approximately 25% of all infants under 1 year of age receive EPSDT vision screening. Approximately 16% of children age 1–5 years are screened. Over 25% of infants under 1 year of age receive hearing screening, and 20% of children age 1–5 receive hearing screening. Figures 3.2–3.5 indicate EPSDT participation overall, and in dental, vision, and hearing screenings.

Figure 3.2. EPSDT Participant Ratio by Age, 1995–1998

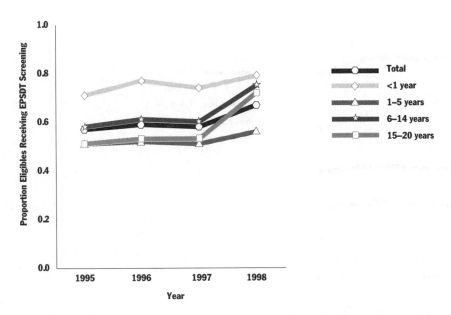

IMMUNIZATIONS

"Baby shots" is the common term for the recommended series of immunizations (also called vaccinations) that are given to infants and children to prevent a variety of diseases. If a young child receives the recommended immunizations, they will be protected against 12 diseases: measles, mumps, rubella (German measles), diphtheria, tetanus (lockjaw), pertussis (whooping cough), polio, Haemophilus influenzae type b (Hib) disease (bacterial infection, usually meningitis), hepatitis A and B, varicella (chicken pox) and pneumococcal disease (Centers for Disease Control and Prevention, 2001a). In 1998, 73% of all children received all immunizations recommended for universal administration (U.S. Department of Health and Human Services, 2000); 77% of all children received the full series for diphtheria, polio, measles-containing vaccine, and Hib disease (see Figure 3.6). Seventy-eight percent of children at or above poverty are fully immunized; 71% of those below the poverty level are immunized (National Immunization Survey, 2001).

SOCIAL AND EMOTIONAL HEALTH

Although we know a lot about how babies are born, how they die, and the status of their physical health, we know very little about another important aspect of development: social and emotional health.

Social and emotional health of infants and toddlers is also known as infant mental health. Infant mental health is the developing capacity of the child from birth to 3 to experience, regulate and express emotions; form close and secure interpersonal relationships; and explore the environment and learn – all in the context of family, community, and cultural expectations for young children (ZERO TO THREE, 2003). Infant mental health is synonymous with healthy social and emotional development.

Figure 3.3. EPSDT Dental Screenings by Age, 1995–1998

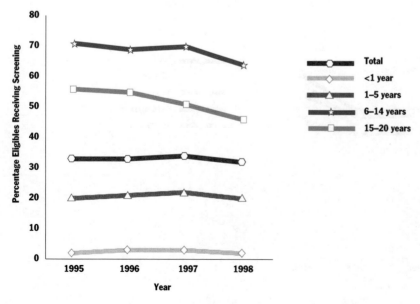

Source: U.S. Department of Health and Human Services Centers for Medicare and Medicaid Services, 2003

Figure 3.4. EPSDT Vision Screenings by Age, 1995–1998

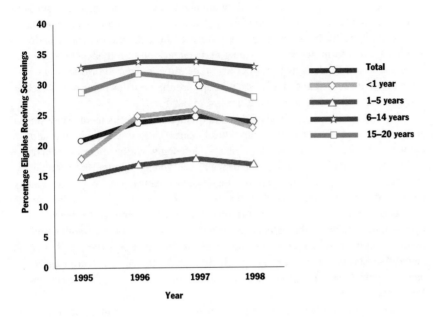

Source: U.S. Department of Health and Human Services Centers for Medicare and Medicaid Services, 2003

Figure 3.5. EPSDT Hearing Screenings by Age, 1995–1998

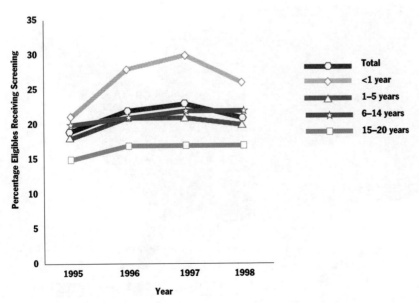

Source: U.S. Department of Health and Human Services Centers for Medicare and Medicaid Services, 2003

Given the importance of social and emotional development in the first 3 years of life, the scarcity of data on the mental health of babies and toddlers is disappointing, but not surprising considering the lack of attention to social and emotional development in infants and toddlers. In the first 3 years, babies and toddlers develop the capacity to form relationships, to give and receive affection, and to express and read emotions. They form the basis for caring and compassion for others, and trust in others. A child's fundamental sense of who they are and what the world is like is established during infancy. Early relationships are the basis for being able to relate and interact with people throughout the rest of our lives.

Most babies experience healthy social and emotional development. They smile and coo, cry and recover, and become social beings. However, some infants and toddlers experience mental health problems. Defining what this means for children under age 3 is not easy. There is still disbelief that young children can even have mental health disorders. There are few highly skilled clinicians to assess the mental health status of infants and toddlers. If there is recognition that infants might have mental health disorders, there is reluctance to label young children for fear of stigmatizing, or of blaming the parents, or for lack of awareness of intervention and treatment options. Although no data are available for children under age 3, it is estimated that between 2% and 8% of all children under the age of 18 are reported to have a mental/emotional problem or functional limitation (Colpe, 2000; Halfon & Newacheck, 1999).

Most parents of young children (72%) believe depression cannot occur until a baby is 1 year old or older. Half of parents of young children (51%) put the age at 3 years or older — higher among dads, lower among moms (DYG, Inc., Civitas, ZERO TO THREE, & Brio, 2000). Research demonstrates that infants begin to experience real depression at about 4 months of age (Luby, 2000)

Chronic maternal depression is associated with less sensitivity in play between mothers and their children during the first 3 years of life; children of women with depressive symptoms performed more poorly on measures of cognitive–linguistic

Figure 3.6. Estimated Immunization Coverage, 2001

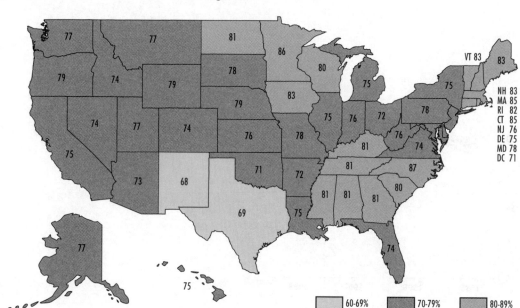

Source: National Immunization Survey, 2001
Note: Children in the 2001 NIS were born between February 1998 and May 2000.

functioning, cooperation, and problem behavior (National Institute of Child Health and Development Early Child Care Research Network, 2001).

SAFETY AND PREVENTION

The number of baby-product injuries to young children decreased almost 20% from 1995 to 1999 (as measured by hospital emergency room visits). This drop was largely attributable to an almost 60% drop in baby walker-related injuries (from 20,100 in 1995 to 8,800 in 1999; Consumer Product Safety Commission, 2000). Deaths due to falls from cribs among infants has also been significantly reduced in recent years, due to more stringent safety standards. Walkers (baby seats on wheels) remain popular with adults, and continue to be a source of injury to infants and toddlers. Educational efforts to reduce the use of walkers have been effective in reducing walker-related falls down stairs by 28% (Conners, Veenema, Kavanaugh, Ricci, & Callahan, 2002). U.S. toy manufacturers may begin widening the base of infant walkers so that they cannot fit through doorways, thereby reducing the number of falls down steps in walkers.

ENVIRONMENTAL ISSUES

The same rapid brain growth that allows a baby to learn so many things in the first 3 years of life also puts the baby's developing brain at risk of being affected by exposure to environmental hazards. Babies and toddlers (and their families) are exposed to a variety of environmental pollutants inside and outside their homes. "Children are more vulnerable to environmental hazards – they breathe more air, drink more water, and eat more food in proportion to their body weight than adults, so they may experience higher rates of exposure" (Population Reference Bureau, 2003b). Mouthing behaviors (infants and toddlers putting objects in their mouths)

Table 3.4. Children's Mental Health Status, Birth to 3, 1990–2000

Percentage of infants and toddlers meeting social–emotional developmental milestones

Milestones	Age birth to 1	Age 1 to 2	Age 2 to 3
Self-regulation			
Interest in surroundings			
Two-way communication			
Problem solving			
Sense of self			
Confidence			
Curiosity			
Socially engaging			
Communicates with others			
Coping strategies to master distress and make transitions			

Source: None

also increase exposure to environmental hazards, especially lead.

Infants and toddlers are involuntarily exposed to cigarette smoke. Tobacco smoke, also known as secondhand smoke, causes low birthweight, chronic middle ear infections, respiratory infections, bronchitis, pneumonia, asthma, and sudden infant death syndrome (SIDS; Centers for Disease Control and Prevention, 2001b). Young children are more susceptible than older children are to the risks of secondhand smoke (National Academy of Sciences, 2000; Dybing & Sanner, 1999).

The number of adults who smoke has decreased over the last decade from 25% overall in 1993 to 22.8% in 2000, and the percentage of homes with children under age 7 in which someone smokes on a regular basis decreased from 29% in 1994 to 19% in 1999. Studies of children exposed to secondhand smoke show that the overall levels of cotinine (a nicotine by-product) in blood samples from children has decreased. A recent report found that 85% of children had detectable levels of cotinine in 1988–1991; between 50 and 75% of children had detectable levels of cotinine in 1999–2000 (U.S. Environmental Protection Agency, 2000).

The metal lead is toxic to the developing brain. Exposure to lead in the environment is known to cause mental retardation and learning disabilities. Lead exposure has also been associated with attention deficit/hyperactivity disorder, hyperactivity and distractibility, higher school dropout rates than for children not exposed to lead, reading disabilities, and increased risk for antisocial and delinquent behavior. In 1999–2000, approximately 300,000 children ages 1–5 years had a blood lead level of 10 micrograms/dL or greater (a level considered elevated). There is no established safe blood lead level — effects on brain development may occur at very low blood lead levels. Blood lead levels in children ages 1–5 have declined by 85% since 1976, primarily due to the phasing out of leaded gasoline between 1973 and 1995 and to reduced numbers of homes with lead-based paint. Lead has also been eliminated from plumbing (including pipes and faucets), food and beverage containers, toys, and playground equipment (U.S. Environmental Protection Agency, 2000)

Table 3.5. Leading Causes of Death in the U.S. for Children Ages 1–4,
         1900 and 2000

1900	Death Rate*
Pneumonia (all forms) and influenza	386.6
Diarrhea, enteritis, and ulceration of the intestines	303.0
Tuberculosis	101.8
2000	
Accidents	12.1
Congenital anomalies	3.3
Cancer	2.8

*Note: Number of deaths per 100,000 children ages 1–4

Source: Population Reference Bureau, 2003a

CHILD FATALITIES

At the beginning of the 20th century, the death rate for infants was much higher than it is today; most deaths were caused by infectious diseases. Prior to World War I, 1 in 10 babies died before the age of 1. The overall death rate in 1900 was 19.8/1,000 children. Today, the overall rate is much lower, at 0.3/1000. The decrease in overall death rate is related to improved standards of living, better sanitation, preventive health care, and availability of antibiotics and immunizations (Population Reference Bureau, 2003a). Table 3.5 compares death rates and leading causes of death in 1990 and 2000.

Accidents (unintentional injuries) are now the leading cause of death in young children. Most unintentional injury deaths among children result from motor vehicle traffic crashes. Motor vehicle deaths are the leading cause of death among children of all ages, and the leading cause of injury-related death among 1–4 year-olds in the United States (National Highway Traffic Safety Administration, 2001). Figures 3.7 and 3.8 display trends in motor vehicle deaths for young children.

Drivers are getting better at restraining young children in car seats. In 2002, 99% of all infants and 94% of all toddlers were restrained in car safety seats, up from 95% and 91%, respectively, in 2000 (Glassbrenner, 2003). The gender gap for drivers using car safety seats for their infant and toddler passengers has all but disappeared. In 2000, 97% of female drivers used car safety seats for child passengers while male drivers used car safety seats 90% of the time. In 2002, 91% of male drivers and 92% of female drivers put their infants and toddlers in car safety seats. Child safety seats have shown to reduce fatal injuries by 71% for infants and by 54% for toddlers.

Home fire is the third highest unintentional (accidental) cause of death for children ages 1 to 4 in the United States. Babies and toddlers are 1.5 times more likely to die in a fire than is general population (U.S. Fire Administration, 2001). Children make up 20% of all fire deaths. Younger children (ages birth through 4) are at a sig-

> **Of the children ages 4 years and younger who were fatally injured in motor vehicle crashes in 2001, nearly 50% were completely unrestrained**
>
> —National Highway Traffic Safety Administration, 2001

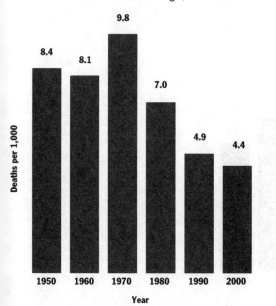

Figure 3.7. Motor Vehicle Deaths, Infants Under 1 Year of Age, 1950–2000

Source: National Center for Health Statistics, 2002a

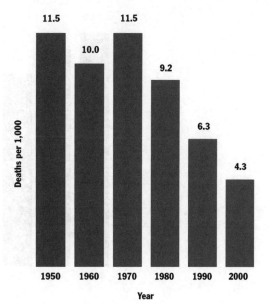

Figure 3.8. Motor Vehicle Deaths, Children Age 1–4 Years of Age, 1950–2000

Source: National Center for Health Statistics, 2002a

nificantly higher risk than older children (5 through 9 years). Although the percentage has decreased from 65% in 1994, babies and toddlers still makes up 60% of all reported fire deaths among children.

Two out of three of the child fire injuries reported each year and three out of four of the child fire deaths each year occurred where there was no operable smoke detector (U.S. Fire Administration, 2001).

BACK TO SLEEP AND TUMMY TO PLAY: IMPACT OF THE BACK TO SLEEP CAMPAIGN ON SUDDEN INFANT DEATH SYNDROME (SIDS) DEATHS

SIDS is the diagnosis given to the sudden death of an infant under 1 year of age that remains unexplained after thorough investigation. SIDS is the leading cause of death in infants between 1 month and 1 year of age. Most deaths occur in babies less than 6 months of age (National Institute of Child Health and Development, 2003). Research indicates that a back-lying sleeping position can lower the risk of SIDS (National Institutes of Health, 2003).

The incidence of SIDS has declined over 50% since 1992 when the American Academy of Pediatrics issued its recommendation that infants should be placed on their back to sleep at all times. The frequency of prone (stomach) sleeping has decreased from greater than 70% in 1992 to approximately 24% of infants in 1996 (American Academy of Pediatrics, 2000a, 2003). Figure 3.9 displays SIDS rates declining from 1980 to 1998.

A national survey of infant sleep practices found variations from state to state. The percentage of respondents who reported putting their babies to sleep on their back was highest in Washington (42.9%) and Alaska (40.8%) and lowest in Georgia (24.5%), Florida (25.4%) and South Carolina (25.8%; Centers for Disease Control and Prevention, 1998a).

Figure 3.9. Annual SIDS Rates, 1980–1998

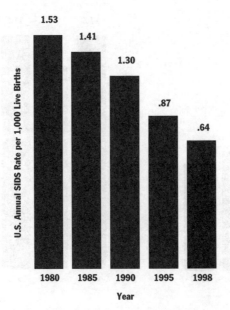

Source: American SIDS Institute (n.d.)

There are also racial differences in back-to-sleep practices. A 10-state study of infant sleeping position found that there is a higher rate of stomach sleeping among African-American babies than among white babies (43% versus 22%) and among some American Indian babies as compared to white babies. For American Indians in two of the states in the study, 16% of respondents in Oklahoma and 33.9% of respondents in Washington reported usually putting babies to sleep on their stomachs. The comparable percentage for Alaska Natives was 23.5% (Centers for Disease Control and Prevention, 1998).

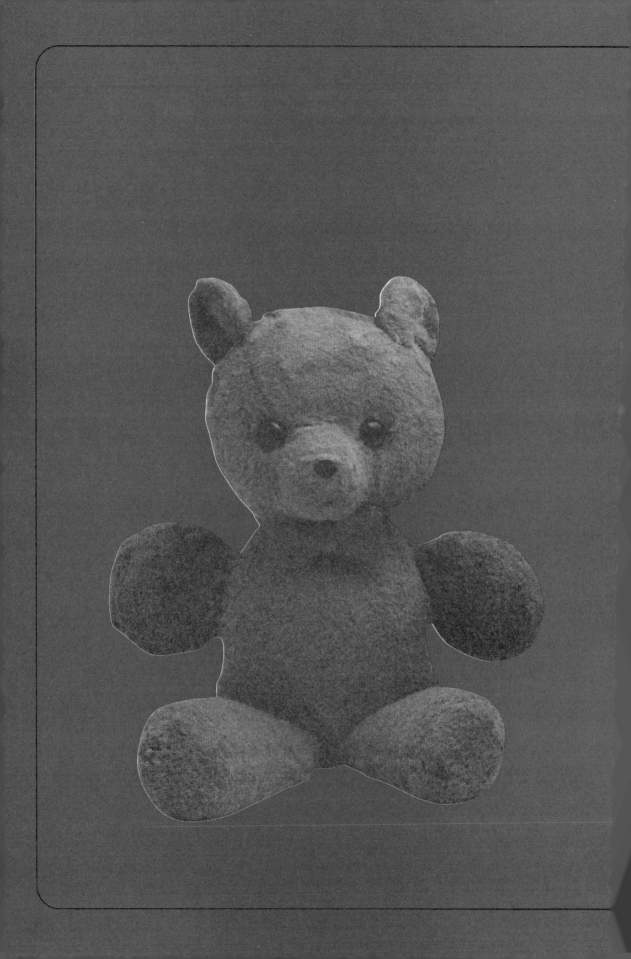

CHAPTER 4
VIOLENCE, TRAUMA,
AND PROTECTIVE SYSTEMS

"The United States is the most violent developed country in the world"

(Osofsky & Fenichel, 2002, p.6).

U nfortunately, exposure to violence is not a new phenomenon for infants and toddlers, but the "threat" of terrorism has become a new reality for young children and families in the United States. In addition to the potential threat of biological and chemical agents, and nuclear, thermonuclear, and mechanical agents, infants and toddlers and their families recently experienced the psychological aspects of terrorism in the September 11, 2001, incidents in New York City, Washington, D.C., and Pennsylvania. There is a heightened awareness of the need to respond to the needs of all children, including infants and toddlers, during disasters.

EXPOSURE TO VIOLENCE

Each year, 3 to 10 million children witness domestic violence (Carter & Stevens, 1999). It is not clear how many infants and toddlers are represented in this number. However, babies can be affected by witnessing violence, as early as 6 months of age. One quarter of parents in a recent national poll have a misconception that young children (6 months or younger) are too young to be affected by witnessing violence because they have no long-term memory (DYG, Inc., et al., 2000). Research shows otherwise.

Children who have been exposed to violence as infants, toddlers, and preschoolers but not referred for intervention until 2 years or more after the incident tend to have significant learning problems, aggressive or withdrawn behavior, and depression. Children who witness violence as early as 2 years of age have memories of the violence (Osofsky, 1997; Osofsky & Dickson, 2000). Infants and toddlers who witness domestic violence show excessive irritability, immature behavior, sleep disturbances, emotional distress, fears of being alone, and regression in toileting and language (Fantuzzo & Mohr, 1999; Osofsky, 1999).

Exposure to violence affects infants and toddlers in several ways depending on the age of the child, the context, the quality of their relationships with parents and other caregivers, previous experience of violence, proximity to the event, and the child's familiarity with the victim or perpetrator (Osofsky, 2000). Even when traumatic events are downplayed by caregivers, young children react to severe trauma with symptoms of posttraumatic stress disorder similar to those seen in adults: sleeplessness, disorganized behavior, and agitation.

Following the attacks in September, 2001, infants and toddlers showed separation anxiety, crying, sleeplessness, rage, and despair. Adults were unaware of just how

Nearly one infant homicide per day was reported in the year 2000—349 total.

—National Center for Injury Prevention and Control, 2000

attuned these very young children were to the parents' and other caregivers' own feelings of loss, shock, numbness, and anger (Schechter, Coates & First, 2001). Even when infants and toddlers are not witnesses to violence, they are deeply affected.

TRAUMA

There were 30,477 violence-related injuries to infants and toddlers reported in 2001 (National Center for Injury Prevention and Control, 2000). Exposure to domestic violence, abuse, and neglect continues for some babies and toddlers. Although the overall rate of violent crime in the United States is decreasing, the rate at which babies under 1 year of age are murdered has risen to the point where it is virtually the same as the homicide rate among adolescents. Twenty-eight babies and toddlers were killed with a gun in 2000 (National Center for Injury Prevention and Control, 2000).

Homicide is the leading cause of injury-related deaths for infants (Brenner, Overpeck, Trumble, DerSimonian & Berendes, 1999). The risk for homicide is greater in infancy than in any other year before age 17. Infants face the greatest risk of homicide on the day they are born. The second-highest period for homicide risk is the eighth week of life, coinciding with the peak age for daily duration of crying in infancy (Barr, 1990). Among homicides on the first day of life, 95% of the victims are not born in a hospital. Infants born to mothers with no prenatal care, less than 12 years of education, two or more previous live births, Native American race, or less than 20 years of age were at twice the risk of injury death compared with the lowest risk groups (Brenner et al., 1999).

A study of 10.7 million births between 1989 and 1991 found that Native American infants are at increased risk for both homicide as well as fatal unintentional injuries while African American infants are at increased risk for homicide, relative to non-Hispanic whites. After controlling for socio-demographic factors, Mexican American infants appear to be protected against both types of injury. Prematurity

> **The perpetrators in shaken baby syndrome are almost always parents or caregivers who shake the baby out of frustration when he is crying inconsolably. Males, either the baby's father or the mother's boyfriend, are the perpetrators in 65%–90% of the cases.**
>
> —Rutherford, 2001

Figure 4.1.
Victimization Rates by Age, Sex, and Maltreatment Type, 2000

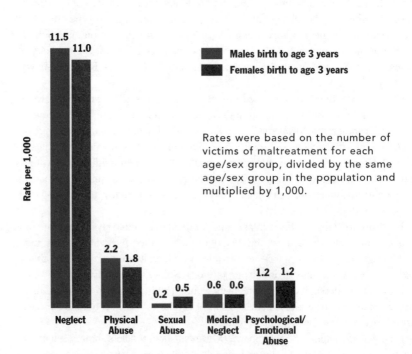

Rates were based on the number of victims of maltreatment for each age/sex group, divided by the same age/sex group in the population and multiplied by 1,000.

Source: US Department of Health and Human Services, Administration for Children and Families, 2002d

and low birth weight are also risk factors for injury-related death. The lower the birth weight, the higher the risk for injury-related death, for both intentional injuries and unintentional injuries (Jain, Khoshnood, Lee & Concato, 2001).

CHILD WELFARE

"Neuroscientific research on early brain development says that young children warranting the greatest concern are those growing up in environments, starting before birth, that expose them to abuse and neglectful care" (Shonkoff & Phillips, 2000, p. 217). Child welfare refers to the field of social services for troubled children and their families. Child welfare services include child protective services, foster care, adoption services, and family preservation and support services (Kamerman, 1998). The federal government gives states leeway in administering and managing their child welfare programs and services. Therefore, there is variation in programs and services from one state to another. The goal of each state's system is the same—to keep children safe and protect them from maltreatment including neglect, physical abuse, sexual abuse, and emotional abuse.

A child's first years of life set the stage for all that follows; future development is based on the experiences and relationships formed during this time. A baby's first attachments to its caregivers are as biologically basic as learning to walk (R. A. Thompson, 2001). Abuse and neglect during the first years yields serious consequences. Separation from parents, sometimes sudden and usually traumatic, coupled with the difficult experiences that have precipitated

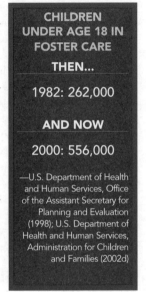

CHILDREN UNDER AGE 18 IN FOSTER CARE

THEN...

1982: 262,000

AND NOW

2000: 556,000

—U.S. Department of Health and Human Services, Office of the Assistant Secretary for Planning and Evaluation (1998); U.S. Department of Health and Human Services, Administration for Children and Families (2002d)

Figure 4.2. Children Birth to Age 5 Years Entering Foster Care, 2000

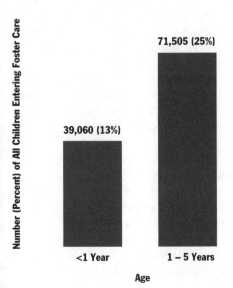

Source: U.S. Department of Health and Human Services, Administration for Children and Families, 2002d

Figure 4.3. Children Birth to Age 5 Years in Foster Care (as of September 30, 2000)

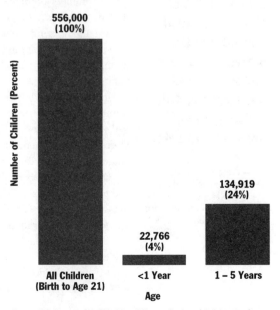

Source: U.S. Department of Health and Human Services, Administration for Children and Families, 2002d

placement in foster care, can leave infants and toddlers impaired in their emotional, social, educational, and physical development. Figure 4.1 displays victimization rates for infants and toddlers.

Infants are the fastest growing category of children entering foster care in the United States, and are likely to stay in care longer than older children (Dicker, Gordon, & Knitzer, 2001; Wulczyn & Hislop, 2002).

Data from the National Multi-state Foster Care Data Archive indicate that 21% of all children in foster care were admitted prior to their first birthday; 45% of all the infant placements occurred within 30 days of the child's birth. These data demonstrate that the high placement rates found for infants are heavily weighted by the experiences of children between birth and 3 months of age (Wulczyn, Hislop & Harden, 2002).

Most of the infants in foster care are placed there because of abuse or neglect that has occurred within the context of parental substance abuse, extreme poverty, mental illness, homelessness, or human immunodeficiency virus (HIV) infection (American Academy of Pediatrics, 2002). They are more likely to have fragile health and disabilities and are far less likely to receive services that address their needs (Dicker et al., 2001; Oser & Cohen, 2003). Infants and toddlers in foster care may show signs of significant delays in language, cognition, and behavior. In fact, they have rates of developmental delay approximately four to five times that found among children in the general population (Dicker & Gordon, 2000).

Multiple, unplanned foster home placements for infants and toddlers may have adverse consequences (American Academy of Pediatrics, 2000b). Early relationships and attachments to a primary caregiver are the most consistent and enduring influence on social and emotional development for very young children (Shonkoff & Philips, 2000). Multiple placements disrupt a child's attachment to primary caregivers and may lead to psychopathology and other problematic outcomes in children (Wulczyn, Kogan, & Harden, in press). With each consecutive placement, a baby has to adjust to a new caregiver and adapt to new routines, rules, and styles of parenting. Babies grieve when their relationships are disrupted. Although children entering foster care as infants experience fewer moves per child than older children, some infants do move three or more times while in foster care (Wulczyn et al., in press). There are no data to clarify why changes in foster care placement are made.

The number of infants and young children entering foster care each year is larger than the number in foster care. When looking at the data for infants in foster care (Figure 4.3), it is important to note that the data represent a count of infants in foster care at a specific point in time (September 30, 2000 for 2000 data) while the data on infants and young children entering foster care (Figure 4.2) represent a cumulative total of all children who entered foster care during the reporting year.

It is difficult to determine whether the infants who entered foster care but not counted on September 30 aged out of the infant age group, whether they were reunified with their parents, or whether they were adopted. It also may be possible that these infants were reunified with their parents and were later returned to foster care and counted under the 1 to 5 age group.

Once they have been removed from their homes and placed in foster care, infants and toddlers are more likely than older children to be abused and neglected and to stay in foster care longer (Wulczyn & Hislop, 2002). Half of the children who were admitted into foster care prior to their first birthday were in care for more than 2 years (26.8 months) while the median duration for children placed before their fourth month of age was the longest, 30.5 months. Older children stayed in care on average for a much shorter time. Children who were between 4 and 17 years of age when they entered foster care stayed in care less than one year (Wulczyn et al., 2002).

Less than 2% of children adopted through the United States foster care system in 1998 were infants; 46% of foreign adoptions were infants.

—Wetzstein, 2002; U.S. Department of Health and Human Services, Administration for Children and Families, 2002c.

Reunification rates are lowest among children who enter placement between birth and 3 months of life: 36% are reunified with their parents compared to 56% of infants who enter foster care at 10–12 months of age (Wulczyn & Hislop, 2002). Although infants and toddlers are less likely than older children to be reunified with their birth parents, they are more likely than older children to be adopted (Wulczyn & Hislop, 2002). When they do return home, they are more likely to experience a recurrence of maltreatment (U.S. Department of Health and Human Services, Administration on Children and Families, 2002a). Figure 4.5 displays fatalities from abuse and neglect.

Of all the children who died from abuse or neglect, 77% were younger than 4 years of age.

—U.S. Department of Health and Human Services, Administration for Children and Families, 2002a.

Figure 4.4. Adoptions From Foster Care, 2000

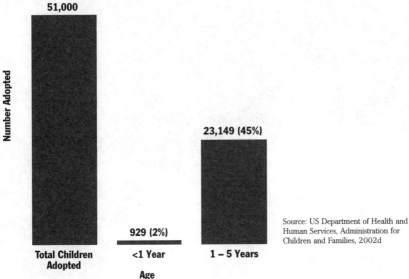

Source: US Department of Health and Human Services, Administration for Children and Families, 2002d

Figure 4.5. Abuse and Neglect Fatalities by Age (Birth to 4 Years), 2000 (as percentage of total number of child deaths from abuse and neglect)

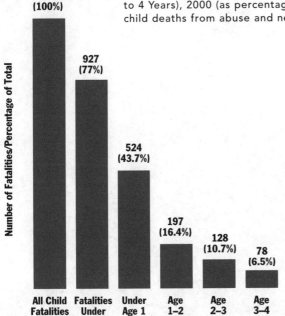

Source: U.S. Department of Health and Human Services, Administration for Children and Families, 2002d.

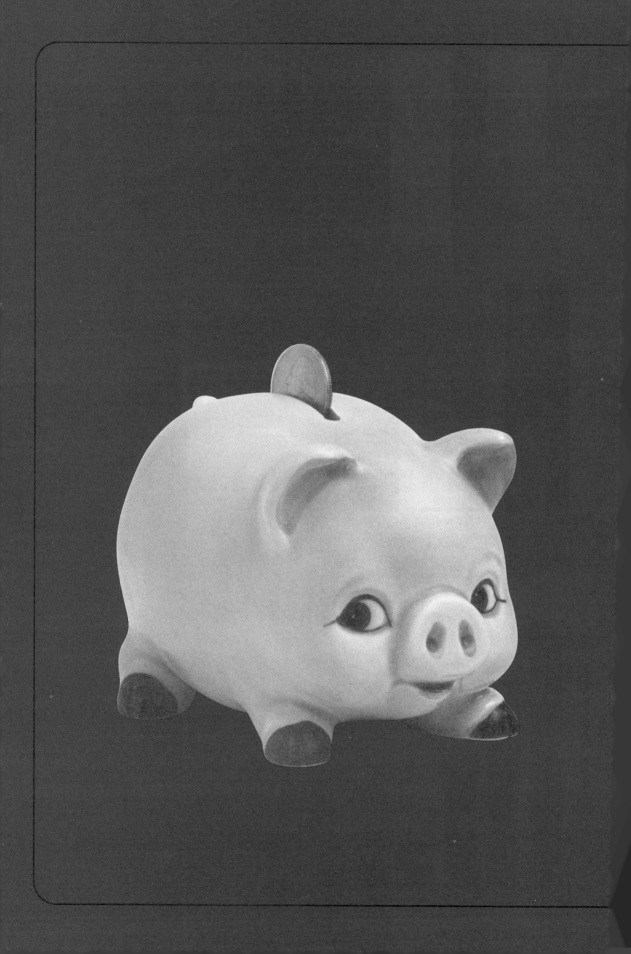

CHAPTER 5
FAMILY AND
ECONOMIC FACTORS

hildren grow and develop in the context of family. Although children gain tremendous independence over the first 3 years of life, they cannot take care of themselves. Infants and toddlers are completely dependent on adults to provide the basics of life: food, shelter, and nurturing. Parents and others who care for babies and toddlers influence their babies' development in many ways every day. Early nurturing experiences such as holding, feeding, and comforting impact the way a baby's brain develops. All parents face the challenge of caring for their children while also taking care of themselves and their other responsibilities. Changes in the nature, schedule, and amount of work by parents of young children, along with economic hardship, make this a tenuous balancing act in spite of higher rates of parental employment (Shonkoff & Phillips, 2000).

This chapter presents data about where and with whom infants and toddlers live. Issues including changes in the ages of parents, marital status, births to teen parents, and the impact of parental education level on child outcomes are discussed. Factors related to the economics of family life are also presented: poverty status, employment, welfare-to-work program participation, and access to health insurance.

FAMILY CHARACTERISTICS

Most—about two thirds—of all babies in the United States are born into husband–wife families. There are over 1 million babies who are born into single-parent families or unmarried two-parent families or who are born and placed in foster care, and eventually adopted. Some single-family homes are headed by fathers, some by mothers (see Figure 5.1).

The number of children under age 18 living with single parents has increased over the past 30 years.

There was a decrease in the number of children living in two-parent households in 2001 (69%) as compared with 1980 (77%; Federal Interagency Forum on Child and Family Statistics, 2002).

Fewer babies are being born to parents who are teenagers. Over the last 10 years, the birth

> **THEN AND NOW:**
>
> THE "TRADITIONAL" FAMILY
>
> 1940: 67% of all married-couple families have a wage-earning dad and a stay-at-home mom.
>
> 1950: 53% of all married-couple families have a wage-earning dad and a stay-at-home mom.
>
> 2000: 16% of all married couple families have a wage-earning dad and a stay-at-home mom.
>
> —Bureau of Labor Statistics, 2003

The percentage of family groups that have four or more children decreased from 17% in 1970 to 6% in 2000.

—Fields & Casper, 2001

Over the river and through the woods: Who lives at Grandma's house?

In 2000, 1,359,000 children under the age of 18 are raised solely by their grandparents.

—American Association of Retired Persons, 2003; American Association for Single People, 2003

rate for females ages 15–19 has continued to drop, reaching a rate of 45.9 births per 1,000 females in 2001.

The adolescent birth rate in 2000 was a record low for the nation at 27 births for every 1,000 young women 15–17 years of age (down from 29 births per 1,000 in 1999). Statistics are not available on teen fathers.

As a percentage of all births, births to mothers under age 18 fell from 6.3% of all births in 1970 to 4.1% in 2000. The most dramatic change in teen birth rate was in births to African-American mothers. Births to African-American mothers under age 18 fell from 14.8% of all births in 1970 to 7.8% in 2000 (see Figure 5.2).

The overall rate of births to unmarried women rose slightly in 2001, while births to unmarried teens declined. About one third of all births in 2001 (33.4%) were to unmarried women (see Figure 5.3 for trend data).

Family composition in the United States has become more varied over the past two decades. A smaller percentage of children lived in two-parent households in 2001 (69%) as compared with 1980 (77%). The percentage of children living with one parent increased from 20% in 1980 to 27% in 1999. Most children who are living with single parents live with a single mother. However, the percentage of children living with single fathers doubled over this time period, from 2% in 1980 to 4% in 1999. Some children live with a single parent who has a cohabiting partner: 16% of children living with single fathers and 9% of children living with single mothers also lived with their parents' partners. There are no precise figures for the number of children under age 3 being raised by gay, lesbian, bisexual, or trans-gendered parents.

Women are waiting longer to have their first child. In 1970, the average age of a mother at the birth of her first baby was 21.4 years; in 2000, it was 24.9 years. Statistics are not available on the average age of a father at birth of his first child (see Figure 5.4).

In 1970, 2,214,000 children under age 18 lived with their grandparents; of these, 957,000 (43%) were being raised solely by their grandparents. In 2000, 3,842,000 children under the age of 18 lived in grandparent-headed households; 1,359,000 (35%) of these children had no parent present in the grandparent-headed household. There are grandparent-headed households in every socioeconomic and ethnic group (American Association of Retired Persons, 2003; American Association for Single People, 2003).

Households with children under age 3 make up about 3% of all households in the United States. Table 5.1 indicates the percentage of households, by region, with infants under age 1.

THEN AND NOW:

SINGLE-PARENT FAMILIES

1970:
7,452,000 children living with mother only (10.8%)
748,000 children living with father only (1.1%)

2000:
16,162,000 children living with mother only (22.4%)
3,058,000 children living with father only (4.2%)

—American Association for Single People, 2003

"FATHERNEED"

Dr. Kyle Pruett defines "fatherneed" as the need in men to provide fathering and the need in their children to experience it (Pruett, 2000, p. 81). Much of the data reported here and in other data books are linked to mother's age, mother's marital status, mother's race — what about the fathers?

Data on fatherhood have yet to become as commonplace in public data

Figure 5.1. Family Households With Children Under Age 3, 2000

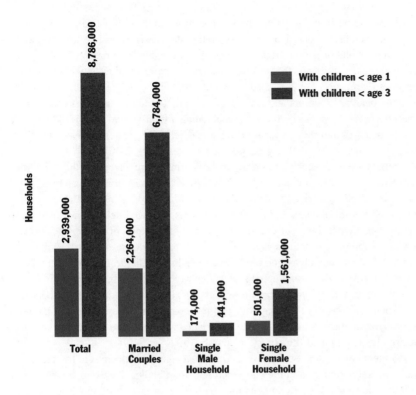

Source: Fields & Casper, 2001

Figure 5.2. Teen Births by Race, 1970–2000

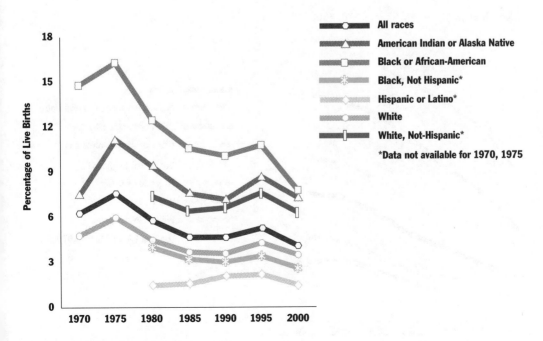

Source: National Center for Health Statistics, 2002a

**Half of all parents
are fathers.**

—Salyers, T., 2003
(personal communication)

**With the exception
of lactation, there
is no evidence that
women are biologi-
cally predisposed
to be better par-
ents than men are.**

—Lamb, 1997, p. 120

sets as maternal characteristics. We don't know, for example, how many fathers are present at the birth of their children, or the educational level of fathers, or the rates of non-marital fatherhood. However, research on fathers is extensive. Studies document father influences on aspects of development ranging from problem-solving abilities, and greater tolerance for stress and frustration, to motor development and gender roles (Lamb, 1997; Lewis, 1997; Nugent, 1991; Pruett, 2000). Fathers also influence the health of mothers and children. One study found that as father involvement levels decrease (from married to non-cohabitating absent), the incidence of low birth weight increases and mother health behaviors deteriorate. Father involvement is strongly related to the mother getting prenatal care (Teitler, 2001).

Fathers are increasingly embracing roles as primary caregivers for their children. In 1996, 18% of children age birth to 5 had their fathers as primary caregivers (Child Trends, 2002). Healthy father involvement has positive effects on child outcomes such as social competence, academic success, reduced delinquency behaviors and personality development that are distinct from the effects of mother–child relationships. Mothers and fathers share many parenting characteristics (such as the desire to feel emotionally connected to one's children, ability to interpret a child's behavioral cues and respond appropriately, anxiety about leaving the child in the care of others, and the predisposition to nurture). However, mothers and fathers also have some differences in the way they approach parenting. These styles are influenced by many factors including culture, social conventions, and the gender of the children being parented (Pruett, 2000; Lamb, 1997).

Mothers have a direct influence on child development outcomes in the prenatal and perinatal period, and in the early months (breastfeeding, for example). One of the indirect maternal influences on child outcomes is maternal educational level. Mother's education level is an important determinant of child outcomes, even more so than family income levels. Maternal education levels have been linked with rates of infant mortality, literacy, and a variety of other competency levels including mathematics, problem solving, communication, perseverance, social skills with peers, social skills

Figure 5.3. Non-Marital Births by Race, 1970–2000

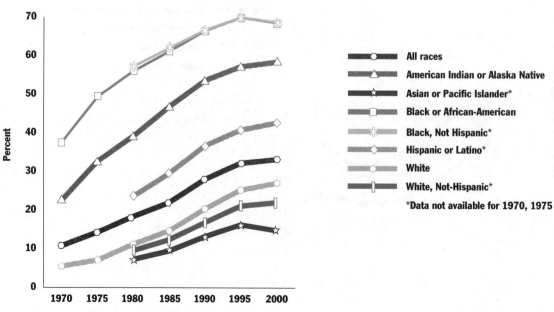

Source: National Center for Health Statistics, 2002a

with adults, individual responsibility, curiosity, and motor skills (Ayoub, Pan, Guinee, & Russell, 2001; Rivers, 2001). In other words, the more formal education the mother has received (high school diploma, college degree, etc.), the better the baby's chances for arriving at school ready to learn. Mothers today are better educated, on the whole, than they were 20 years ago (see Figure 5.5).

Figure 5.4. Non-Marital Births by Age of Mother, 1970–2000

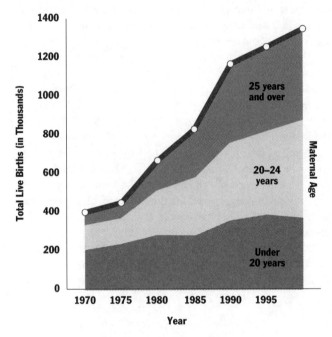

Source: National Center for Health Statistics, 2002a

Table 5.1. Distribution of Families With Infants, by Region, 2000

WHERE DO FAMILIES WITH INFANTS UNDER 1 YEAR OF AGE LIVE?

Region	Number of households with children under age 1	Percentage of all households	All households
Northeast	591,000	3	20,087,000
South	1,177,000	3	37,303,000
Mid-West	839,000	3	24,508,000
West	818,000	4	22,808,000

Source: U.S. Census Bureau, 2001

FAMILIES IN THE MILITARY

As this book goes to press, thousands of U. S. troops remain stationed in Iraq and Afghanistan. The troops deployed there, and in other areas of the world, as well as those who are maintaining the military structure within the United States, include many parents of infants and toddlers.

Policymakers at the Office of Children and Youth, Department of Defense, keep abreast of current trends in early care and education, issues impacting military families, and factors impacting the demand for care through the Military Family Resource Center (MFRC). MFRC is a tool for enhancing the effectiveness of military family policy and programs. MFRC's mission is to act as a catalyst of information between the Department of Defense Military Community and Family Policy (MCFP) office, military policymakers, and program staff, and to deliver timely, efficient, and effective information services through cutting-edge technology.

The Department of Defense reports information about Active Duty families in all branches of military (Army, Navy, Marine Corps, Air Force) as well as families in the Selected Reserves (Army National Guard, Army Reserve, Naval Reserve, Marine Corps Reserve, Air National Guard, Air Force Reserve, and Coast Guard Reserve).

In 2002, there were 1,402,120 Active Duty military members with 1,916,056 family members. In the Selected Reserves, there were 882,142 military members with 1,076,663 family members (Thompson, in press). Less than half of Active Duty military members have children (defined as age 23 or under). Over one third of Active Duty members (37.7%) are married with children and a small percent (6.4%) are single parents. In the Selected Reserves, over one third (34.4%) of members have children. Over one quarter of the Selected Reserves (28.1%) are married with children, and a small percentage (6.3%) are single parents.

Many military parents are parents of infants and toddlers (see Table 5.2). Among Active Duty Military, 33,433 members gave birth to their first child in 2001. In the Select Reserves, 4,365 members had their first child in 2001. Although precise figures

Figure 5.5. Births by Mother's Education Level

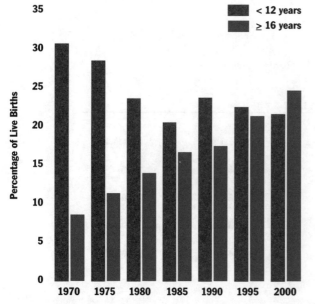

Source: National Center for Health Statistics, 2002a

Table 5.2. Infants and Toddlers in Military Families, 2001

Active Duty Family	**318,242 children under age 3**
Select Reserve Families	**83,290 children under age 3**
Total all children birth to 3	**401,532 children**

Source: Thompson, in press

are not available, it is probable that many of these military members are deployed in 2003.

"The Department of Defense military child development system provides services for the largest number of children on a daily basis of any employer in the United States" (Military Family Resource Center, 2003, p. 1). The Department of Defense views child care as an issue that impacts the effectiveness and readiness of the military workforce. Over 1.2 million children total, including 244,000 children under the age of 3, are served in the military child care environment (Military Family Resource Center, 2003).

Congress passed the Military Child Care Act in 1989. The goal of this legislation was to improve availability, quality, safety, and management of child care provided on military installations. The Military Child Care Act required changes in child care provision in all branches of the military. Major changes included an increase in the military's mandated contribution to the operation of Child Development Services; development of training materials and requirements for child care staff; pay increases for child care employees at rates equivalent to that of other employees with comparable training, seniority, and experience on the same military installation; employment preference for military spouses; uniform parent fees based on family income; expanded child abuse prevention and safety; establishing parent boards; at each center; a study of child care demand; subsidies for family home day care, and a demonstration program for accreditation of military child development programs (RAND, 1998; RAND, 2003). After implementing changes in provider wages, accreditation standards, inspections, and oversight procedures, the military child care system is now considered a model for the nation.

FAMILY EXPENSES AND ECONOMIC STABILITY

Raising children is an expensive proposition. Estimated expenses for raising infants and toddlers vary considerably by household income level. According to the U.S. Department of Agriculture, depending on the age of the child, annual child-rearing expenses range from $6,490 to $7,560 for families in the lowest income group, from $9,030 to $10,140 for families in the middle-income group, and from $13,410 to $14,670 for families in the highest income group. Table 5.3 lists the total cost of raising a child from birth to age 18.

It generally costs more to raise young children in the urban West, followed by the urban Northeast and urban South. It costs the least to raise young children in the urban Midwest and rural areas of the United States.

Mean family incomes are higher for white families with children than for African-American and Hispanic families with children. In 1995, for example, white families had family incomes that were about 65% higher than African-American families, and 71% higher than Hispanic families. Among husband–wife families, the white–African-American disparity is smaller, with whites having incomes that

> **The average baby uses between 7,000 and 9,000 disposable diapers ($2,000 worth) before being potty trained.**
>
> —McConnell, 1998

THEN AND NOW: MEAN FAMILY INCOME		
	1980	**1995**
All families	$44,015	$50,161
Married-couple families	$49,846	$50,161
Female head of household, No husband present	$19,555	$21,905

—U.S. Department of Health and Human Services, 1997

are 16% higher. The disparity between whites and Hispanics remains almost as large for husband–wife families, however, with white families having average incomes 61% higher than their Hispanic counterparts.

Spending patterns for child-rearing expenses are similar for single-parent and husband–wife households. The difference is that most single-parent households are in the lower income group. Single-parent households with two children spend, on average, $5,440 each year on their babies and toddlers. Husband–wife families spend an average of $6,490 on the babies and toddlers in the family (Lino, 2002).

Housing accounts for the largest portion of family expenses, at 33% to 37% of all expenses. Food is the next largest expenditure for families, regardless of income level, accounting for 15% to 20% of child-rearing expenses (Lino, 2002). Child care and educational expenses for babies and toddlers represent 2–3% of a family's overall cost of raising their children.

FAMILIES WITHOUT HOMES

Although no specific data are available for homeless families who have children under age 3, families with children account for 40% of the homeless population (National Coalition for the Homeless, 2002).

One of the fastest growing segments of the homeless population is families with children. Families with children constitute approximately 40% of people who become homeless (Silver & Pañares, 2000). A survey of 30 U.S. cities found that in 1998, children accounted for 25% of the homeless population (U.S. Conference of Mayors, 1998). These proportions are likely to be higher in rural areas; research indicates that families, single mothers, and children make up the largest group of people who are homeless in rural areas (Vissing, 1996).

WORKING FAMILIES

Most children under age 3 have working parents. The percentage of working mothers has changed over the last three decades. In 1970, 24% of mothers with children under age 2 were employed. By 1984, the percentage had risen to 46.8%. In 2000, 60.4% of mothers of children under age 3 were employed (U.S. Department of Labor Current Population Survey, 2002). Much of this increase can be attributed to the growth in the number of children living with working single mothers, which rose from 33% in 1993 to 50% in 2000. Fewer mothers with infants were employed full time (60.8%) than were mothers without infant children (76.9%) (Bachu & O'Connell, 2000).

In married-couple households in which both the husband and wife are employed (either full time or part time), over 25% of the women earned more money in 1999 than did their husbands the previous year. In households in which both the husband and the wife are employed full time, the number of women earning more than their husbands increases to 31% (Population Reference Bureau, 2003b).

In spite of the increase in the number of working parents, especially working mothers, poverty remains a problem for families of infants and toddlers; 2.8 million babies and toddlers are poor. The poverty rate for children living with family members in 1999 and 2000 was reported to be at its lowest rate since 1979. The decrease in poverty was most evident in families headed by women, and was more pronounced for African-American children (Federal Interagency Forum on Child and Family Statistics, 2002). Table 5.4 describes poverty rates by age and race/ethnicity for infants and toddlers.

Americans throw away 49 million diapers per day. Today's diapers will still be in landfills 300 years from now.

—McConnell, 1998

The typical homeless family is a single mother in her 20's with two children under the age of six.

—Homes for the Homeless, 2003

Table 5.3. What it Costs to Raise a Child, Birth to 18 Years (Based on 2001, Before-Tax Income)

Lower income families (less than $39,100 annual income)	$124,800
Middle income families ($35,100 to $65,800)	$170,460
Higher income families (more than $65,800)	$249,180

Source: Lino, 2002.

Mom always liked you better!

In single-parent households with two children, about 7% less is spent on the older child than on the younger child at a specific age category.

—Source: Lino, 2002

Table 5.4 Infants and Toddlers Living in Poverty*, 2000 (numbers in thousands)

	TOTAL	BELOW POVERTY LEVEL	
		Number	Percentage
All groups, all ages	275,924	31,054	11.3
All groups			
Age <1 year	3,836	977	25.5
1 Year	4,002	966	24.1
2 Years	3,921	896	22.8
Total 0–3	11,759	2,839	24.1
White			
Age <1 year	3,093	691	22.3
1 Year	3,068	605	19.7
2 Years	3,080	590	19.2
Total 0–3	9,241	1,886	20.4
African-American			
Age <1 year	547	236	43.1
1 Year	693	304	43.8
2 Years	591	253	42.8
Total 0–3	1,831	793	43.2
Hispanic			
Age <1 year	801	361	45.0
1 Year	704	281	39.9
2 Years	716	278	38.8
Total 0–3	2,221	920	41.2
White, Non-Hispanic			
Age <1 year	2,318	341	14.7
1 Year	2,405	346	14.4
2 Years	2,408	330	13.7
Total 0–3	7,131	1017	14.3

*Poverty = annual income of $14,128 for a family of three in 2001.
Source: U.S. Bureau of Labor Statistics Current Population Survey (2001b).

TEMPORARY ASSISTANCE FOR NEEDY FAMILIES (TANF)[1]

Under TANF, the federal government provides funds to states in the form of a block grant. States are able to use their TANF funds in any manner "reasonably calculated to accomplish the purposes of TANF." The four key purposes outlined in Public Law 104-193 are to:

- provide assistance to needy families so that children can be cared for in their own homes or in homes of relatives;
- end dependence of needy parents on government benefits by promoting job preparation, work, and marriage;
- prevent and reduce incidence of out-of-wedlock pregnancies; and
- encourage the formation and maintenance of two-parent families.

States have been using their funds in a variety of ways including: cash assistance, child care, education and job training, transportation, and a variety of other services to help families make the transition to work. In 2001, 18% of the total state TANF funding was used for child care (Parrott & Neuberger, 2002). Between fiscal year 1992 and fiscal year 2001, the percentage of families participating in TANF with a youngest child who was a toddler (i.e., between age 1 and 2) declined from 30% to 20%. At the same time, the percentage of families whose youngest child was age 6 or older increased from 36% to 45% of all TANF families with children (U.S. Department of Health and Human Services, Administration for Children and Families, 2003a). See Table 5.5 for changes in TANF enrollment for infants and toddlers.

TANF gives states the option of not requiring a single custodial parent caring for a child under age 1 to engage in work. Although TANF gives states this option, just over half the states take advantage of this opportunity. As of June 1, 2001, states used the following child age criteria to exempt parents from work requirements:

- 4 states have an exemption for families with a youngest child over 12 months of age (ranging from 18 months to 6 years);
- 23 states exempt families with a child under the age of 12 months from work requirements;
- 19 states exempt families with a child under the age of 6 months from work requirements;
- 4 states do not have an automatic age of youngest child exemption and make their decisions on a case-by-case basis.
- 1 state responded "not applicable" as their counties have discretion to provide exemptions from work requirements (U.S. Department of Health and Human Services, Administration for Children and Families, 2003a).

HEALTH INSURANCE

Sixty percent of children in the United States are covered under private health insurance provided through a parent's employer (Hoffman & Wang, 2003). Changes in the economy usually affect family income as well as insurance coverage for the adults and the children in the household. Between 2000 and 2001, the number of people in low-income families increased by 3.1 million and the number of people with higher

---

[1] Temporary Assistance to Needy Families (TANF; 42 U.S.C. section 607(b)(5), a federal program enacted in 1996 under the Personal Responsibility and Work Opportunity Reconciliation Act, established the federal income assistance program for families in poverty. TANF replaced the Aid to Families with Dependent Children (AFDC) program, which provided cash welfare to poor children and their families since 1935.

incomes decreased by 700,000. During the same time, there was a decrease in the number of children and adults covered by employer-sponsored private insurance. The number of uninsured children would have grown even more but states made concerted efforts to enroll more children in Medicaid and State Children's Health Insurance Programs (SCHIP)[2].

Between 2000 and 2001, the number of children covered by employer-sponsored health insurance dropped by 0.9% for the poor, 2.8% for the near poor (incomes at 100%–199% of poverty), and 1.1% for those children in higher income families. During the same time period, the number of children covered by Medicaid, SCHIP and other state programs, Medicare, and military-related programs grew by 1.4% for children in poverty, 2.8% for the near-poor, and 0.9% for children in homes with higher income. A higher percentage of infants under age 1 are uninsured as compared to all children under age 19.

Nationwide, 12.9% of all infants under age 1 and 10.3% of all children under age 5 are uninsured (Hoffman and Wang, 2003). Among children whose families make less than 200% of the poverty level, numbers are higher: 18.4% of these infants are uninsured, and 16.6% of all children in families with low incomes under age 5 are uninsured. Tables 5.6–5.8 describe health insurance status of infants and young children.

---

[2] State Children's Health Insurance Program (SCHIP): In 1997, Congress passed the Balanced Budget Act of 1997, which established the State Children's Health Insurance Program (SCHIP). This program was designed to expand health insurance coverage for uninsured children in families with low incomes, up to 200% of the federal poverty level. SCHIP gives states the option of using Medicaid, or some combination of SCHIP and Medicaid, to expand coverage for eligible children. In fiscal year 2001, 4.6 million children (up to age 19) were covered under SCHIP.

Table 5.5. Children Age Birth to 3 Years Receiving AFDC/TANF, 1992–2000

	1992	1996	2000
Unborn	2.0%	1.5%	0.6%
Age birth–1 year	10.3%	10.4%	13.3%
Age 1-2 years	29.7%	24.3%	19.9%

Source: 2002 TANF Annual Report to Congress, U.S. Department of Health and Human Services, Administration for Children and Families, 2003a.

Table 5.6. Health Insurance Coverage of Children Ages 1–5, 2001

	Children (million)	Private		Public		Uninsured
		Employer	Individual	Medicaid	Other	
Total all children (under age 19)	76.6	59.9%	4.1%	22.3%	1.6%	12.1%
<1 year of age	3.9	52.6%	2.5%	29.7%	2.3%	12.9%
1-5 year of age	19.5	57.4%	3.0%	27.8%	1.6%	10.3%

Distribution by Coverage Type

Source: Hoffman & Wang, 2003

Table 5.7. Health Insurance Coverage of Children From Families With Low Incomes
(Less Than 200% of Poverty), Ages 1–5, 2001

| | Children in families with low incomes (millions) | Distribution by Coverage Type | | | | |
| | | Private | | Public | | Uninsured |
		Employer	Individual	Medicaid	Other	
Total low income children (under age 19)	31.9	28.6%	3.6%	44.7%	1.7%	21.3%
<1 year of age	1.9	21.5%	1.9%	55.0%	3.2%	18.4%
1-5 year of age	8.9	27.6%	2.0%	51.9%	1.9%	16.6%

Source: Hoffman & Wang, 2003

Table 5.8. Characteristics of Uninsured Children Ages 1–5, 2001

	Children (millions)	Percentage of children	Uninsured (millions)	Percentage of uninsured	Uninsured rate
Total all children (under age 19)	76.6	100	9.2	100	12.1%
<1 year of age	3.9	5.1	0.5	5.5	12.9%
1-5 year of age	19.5	25.5	2.0	21.6	10.3%

Source: Hoffman & Wang, 2003

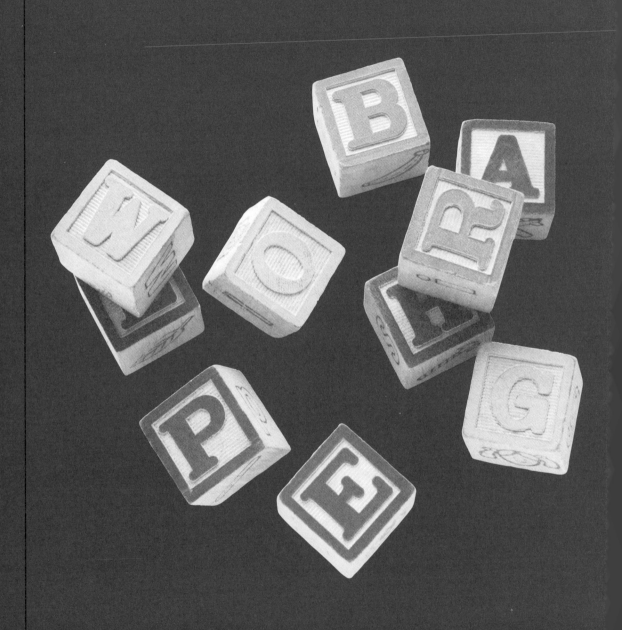

CHAPTER 6
EARLY LEARNING AND CARE

he first 3 years of life are a period of extraordinary growth — physical, intellectual, social, emotional, and linguistic growth. During this time, the brain undergoes its most rapid development, and most infants and toddlers begin to think, feel, speak, learn, and make choices.

Both nature and nurture affect brain development. Chapters 2–5 discuss factors that can influence brain development. Genetic factors, birth conditions, early experiences and relationships, exposure to injury and toxins in the environment, and family support and stability all have an impact on a child's developmental journey. No single factor is responsible for determining a child's developmental outcome. No single activity or intervention, by itself, can "inoculate" a child from future trauma or guarantee a happy, healthy, productive life. It is the interaction of nature and nurture that help to promote resilience, protect from harm, and reduce risk to the child's early development.

From the first moments of life, babies are "wired to learn." The learning that takes place in the first years of life lays the foundation for future school and life success (Shonkoff & Phillips, 2000). The goal of ensuring that all children enter school "ready to learn" has become a national priority. Research demonstrates that high-quality comprehensive services for at-risk families with young children can improve children's life outcomes. As they grew up, the children who attended high-quality early childhood programs showed a reduced need for special education, improved high school graduation rates, fewer arrests, higher earnings, and higher home ownership than children who did not receive a high-quality early childhood experience. The return on investment for early childhood programs more than pays for initial start-up and program maintenance costs.

'Itsy Bitsy (aka 'Eentsy Weentsy') Spider' is the favorite song of America's babies and toddlers and has been for two generations.

—Johnson-Green & Custodero, 2002, p. 47

EARLY LITERACY

Increasingly, the goal of assuring that children are ready for school is a national priority. School readiness and early literacy are sometimes viewed as one and the same. Early literacy is, however, only one part of what makes a child school ready. Early (or emergent) literacy is what children know about reading and writing before they can actually read and write. It encompasses all the experiences that children have had with books, language, and print, beginning in infancy. Because these experiences unfold in the context of relationships, they are linked to, and dependent on, social–emotional development.

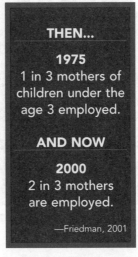

THEN...

1975
1 in 3 mothers of children under the age 3 employed.

AND NOW

2000
2 in 3 mothers are employed.

—Friedman, 2001

A national survey reports that 52% of parents said they read stories every day with their children ages 4 to 35 months. Even more parents of infants and toddlers (age 4 to 35 months) play music or sing songs with their child every day (Halfon et al., in press). An earlier survey reported that 39% of children under age 3 were read to each day (U.S. Department of Education, 1999). Only 4%–5% of adults are unable to read a children's book, although more may be uncomfortable doing so (U.S. Department of Education, 1999).

Early literacy evolves from a number of earlier behaviors and skills including book handling; looking at books and recognizing pictures; imitating actions in a picture or talking about the events in a story; babbling in imitation of reading; running fingers along printed words; and learning rhythms of language through storytelling, singing, and clapping (Schickedanz, 1999).

CHILD CARE

> **39% of babies and toddlers are in child care 35 or more hours per week.**
>
> —Ehrle, Adams, & Tout, (2001).

The majority of children under age 3 have working parents and spend a significant amount of time in non-parental child care (see Figures 6.2 and 6.4). Each day, an estimated 6 million children under age 3 spend some or all of their day being cared for by someone other than their parents (Ehrle, Adams, & Tout, 2001). With the increase in the workforce of the number of mothers with babies and toddlers, the need for quality child care has become even more critical. Child care enables parents to return to work, stay employed, or attend school — all of which contribute to the economic security and livelihood of young families. See Figure 6.1 for changes in maternal employment over the past 25 years. The lack of quality child care that exists for babies and toddlers is a major barrier to employment. According to a recent study conducted by ZERO TO THREE and Mathematica Policy Research, families with low incomes who have infants and toddlers face numerous barriers to accessing good-quality child care including: inadequate supply of infant–toddler care, lack of

Figure 6.1. Trends in Employment for Mothers of Young Children (as a percentage of all mothers in the workforce with children)

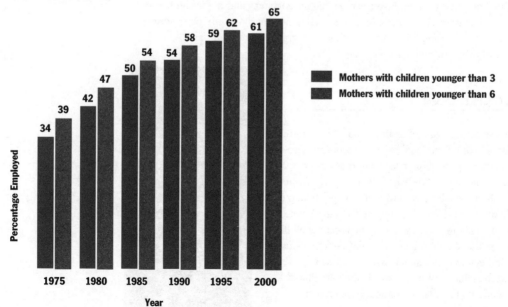

Legend:
- Mothers with children younger than 3
- Mothers with children younger than 6

Source: Phillips & Adams, 2001.

high-quality infant–toddler child care, the high cost of infant–toddler child care, difficulties accessing and maintaining child care subsidies, and lack of transportation (Paulsell, Nogales, & Cohen, 2003).

Many more mothers of young children are employed now than 25 years ago, and more infants and toddlers are spending significant amounts of time in non-parental

Figure 6.2. Regulated Child Care in the United States, 2002

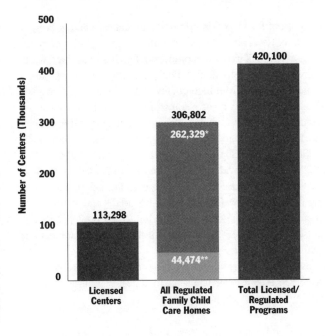

Note: Includes data from the 50 states, District of Columbia, Puerto Rico, and the Virgin Islands. The majority of these programs serve infants and toddlers as well as older children. Center data include some 2001 reporting.

* **Regulated small family child care homes**
** **Regulated group family child care homes**

Source: Martin, Hamilton, Ventura, Menacher, & Park, 2002

Figure 6.3. Primary Child Care Arrangements for Children Under Age 3 With Employed Mothers

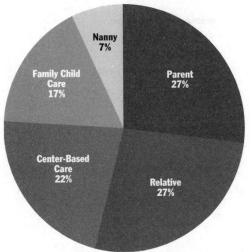

Source: Ehrle, Adams, & Tout, (2001).

care (see Figure 6.2). Second only to the immediate family, child care is the context in which early development unfolds for most of our nation's babies and toddlers (Shonkoff & Phillips, 2000). The science of early childhood development demonstrates the importance of early experiences, noting that early care has a long-lasting impact on how young children develop, on their ability to learn, and on their capacity to regulate their own emotions (Shonkoff & Phillips, 2000). Babies learn and take their cues from the adults around them — their parents, their child care providers, and other important adults in their daily lives. Early exposure to supportive, nurturing child care provides babies with a template that helps them navigate through each new experience with confidence and success.

Quality child care is important for all children in non-parental care and is even more critical for at-risk children. Research indicates that the strongest effects of quality child care are found with at-risk children — children from families with the fewest resources and under the greatest stress (Shonkoff & Phillips, 2000). Yet, at-risk babies and toddlers who may benefit the most from high-quality child care are the least likely to receive it. These infants and toddlers receive some of the poorest quality care that exists in communities across the United States. The poor quality that they receive may diminish inborn potential and will lead to poorer cognitive, social, and emotional developmental outcomes (Shonkoff & Phillips, 2000). A national study of 100 child care centers found that 92% of them provided inadequate care to babies. According to the study, these centers did not meet children's needs for health, safety, nurturing relationships, and learning (Cost, Quality & Child Outcomes Study Team, 1995).

The number of regulated child care centers increased in 2003 by 2.7% to a total of 116,409 centers (see Figure 6.3). The majority of them care for infants and toddlers, in addition to children over age 3.

The average annual cost of center care for an infant in an urban area ranges from $3,900 in Arkansas to $12,978 in Massachusetts. In almost two thirds of the

> **Poor families who paid for child care spent roughly three times more of their budget than non-poor families on child care (20% compared with 7%)**
>
> —Smith, 2002, p. 17.

Figure 6.4. Primary Child Care Arrangements for Children Under Age 3 With Employed Mothers (by Child's Age and Family Structure)

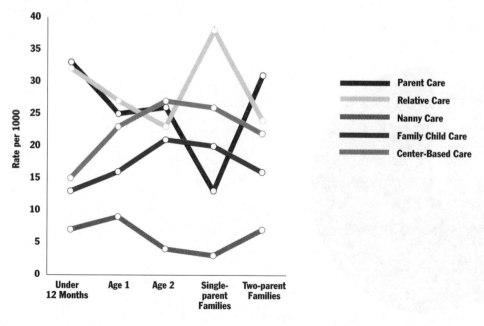

Source: Ehrle, Adams, & Tout (2001).

states, the average annual cost is over $5,750. The average cost is over $6,750 per year in more than one third of the states (Schulman, 2002).

Child care workers are not highly paid. The average hourly wage for a center-based child care worker is $8.91 (U.S. Bureau of Labor Statistics, 2001a). Low wages may contribute to high turnover rates. Of the child care centers surveyed in 1996, 75% of all teaching staff and 40% of the center directors were no longer on the job when centers were visited again in 2000 (Whitebrook, Sakai, Gerber, & Howes, 2001).

FEDERAL SUPPORT FOR CHILD CARE: THE CHILD CARE AND DEVELOPMENT FUND

The Personal Responsibility and Work Opportunity Reconciliation Act of 1996 revamped the structure of federal funding for child care and created the Child Care and Development Fund (CCDF). This block grant allows states flexibility in administering child care programs and establishes a single set of rules and regulations that apply to all components of the fund. The CCDF has three funding streams: mandatory, discretionary, and matching. States are required to spend a minimum of 4% of CCDF funds on activities designed to improve the quality of child care. Figure 6.5 shows the percentage of children served through CCDF.

Currently, $100 million of the federal CCDF funds are earmarked for strategies to increase the supply and improve the quality of child care for infants and toddlers. This infant–toddler set-aside, currently earmarked through the appropriations process, has helped states to invest in specialized infant–toddler provider training, to provide technical assistance to programs and practitioners, and to link compensation with training and demonstrated competence.

Early Head Start serves 70,000 babies, toddlers, and pregnant women through 708 community-based programs, only 3% of the eligible population.

—U.S. Department of Health and Human Services, Administration for Children and Families, 2002a

Figure 6.5. Child Care Development Fund—Children Served by Age Group, 2001

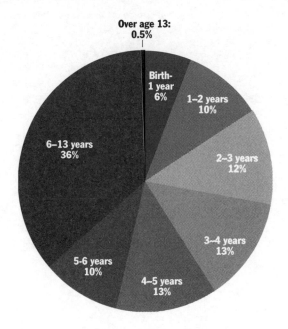

Source: US Department of Health and Human Services, Administration for Children and Families, 2003a

HIGHLIGHTS FROM THE NATIONAL EVALUATION OF EARLY HEAD START

INTELLECTUAL, SOCIAL, AND EMOTIONAL DEVELOPMENT

• **Early Head Start Moves Children Further Along the Path that Could Lead to Greater School Readiness if the Early Head Start Gains are Maintained by Good-Quality Preschool Programs.** Early Head Start produced statistically significant, positive impacts on standardized measures of children's cognitive and language development. A smaller percentage of Early Head Start children (27.3 % versus 32%) scored in the "at-risk" range of developmental functioning (although still below the mean of national norms). By keeping children from entering the lowest-functioning group, Early Head Starting may be reducing the risk of later poor cognitive, language, and school outcomes.

• **Early Head Start Children Had More–Positive Interactions With Their Parents** than control group children. Positive and secure parent–child relationships may reduce a young child's fear in novel or challenging situations and enable the child to explore with confidence.

• **Early Head Start Children Were More Attentive to Objects During Play** than control group children. Play is important because being attentive to and engaged in play activities is how children begin to learn important cognitive and social skills needed for later school and life success.

PARENTING AND FAMILIES

• **Early Head Start Parents Were More Involved and Provided More Support for Learning.** Early Head Start programs have significant favorable impacts on a range of parenting outcomes. Early Head Start parents were observed to be more emotionally supportive and less detached than control-group parents. They also provided significantly more support for language and learning than control-group parents.

• **Early Head Start Helped Parents Move Toward Self-Sufficiency.** Early Head Start significantly facilitated parents' progress toward self-sufficiency. Although there were not significant increases in income, there was increased parental participation in education and job-training activities.

• **Early Head Start Programs Had a Substantial Impact on African American Families and a Favorable Pattern of Impacts on Hispanic and White Families.** Early Head Start programs were especially effective in improving child development and parenting outcomes of African American children and parents. The Early Head Start programs also had a favorable pattern of impacts on Hispanic and white children and parents.

• **Early Head Start Had Favorable Impact on Child–Father Interactions.** Early Head Start significantly improved how fathers interacted and related to their children. Early Head Start children were observed to be more able to engage their fathers and to be more attentive during play than control group children. Early Head Start fathers were observed to be less intrusive in interacting with their children than control group fathers. The emotional quality of the father–child relationship appears to be extremely important to children's adjustment and well-being.

• **Early Head Start Participation Resulted in Fewer Subsequent Births.** Mothers in Early Head Start were less likely to have subsequent births within the 2 years following enrollment in Early Head Start.

Source: ZERO TO THREE Policy Center, 2003

EARLY HEAD START

All babies and toddlers need positive early learning experiences to foster their intellectual, social, and emotional development and to lay the foundation for later school success. Babies and toddlers living in high-risk environments need additional supports to promote their healthy growth and development. Disparities in children's cognitive and social abilities become evident well before they enter Head Start or pre-kindergarten programs at age 4. Early Head Start (EHS) was created in 1995 with bipartisan support to intervene earlier in the lives of at-risk babies and toddlers, minimizing these disparities and ensuring that children enter school ready to learn.

EHS is the only federal program specifically designed to improve the early education experiences of infants and toddlers from families with low incomes. The goals of EHS are: to promote healthy prenatal outcomes for pregnant women; to enhance the development of very young children; and to promote healthy family functioning. Research from the national evaluation of EHS — a rigorous, large-scale, random-assignment evaluation — concluded that EHS is making a positive difference in areas associated with children's success in school, family self-sufficiency, and parental support of child development. What is most compelling about the EHS data is that they reflect a broad set of indicators that show positive impacts on enrollees. Patterns of impacts varied in meaningful ways for different subgroups of families.

Figure 6.6 and Table 6.1 describe program enrollment and funding. It should be noted that Figure 6.6 reports all enrollees in EHS for FY2002 plus participants who

Figure 6.6. Growth of EHS, Enrollees and Funding, Federal Fiscal Years 1995–2002

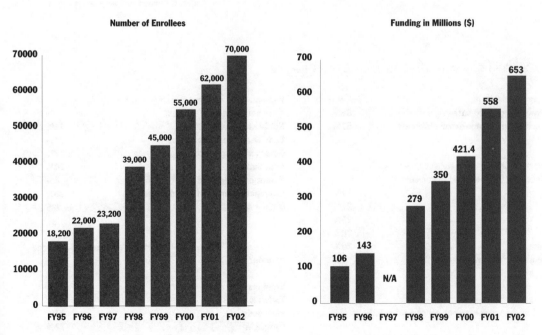

Source: J. Jerald, Personal Communication, March 21, 2003

Table 6.1. EHS Programs by State and Number Served, 2001–2002

State	#of Programs	#of Children Enrolled	State	#of Programs	#of Children Enrolled	State	#of Programs	#of Children Enrolled
Alabama	7	531	Kentucky	11	1177	Ohio	19	1782
Alaska	3	401	Louisiana	11	664	Oklahoma	8	968
Arizona	6	847	Maine	5	434	Oregon	8	895
Arkansas	8	711	Maryland	12	1101	Pennsylvania	26	2893
California	50	6993	Massachusetts	10	902	Puerto Rico	13	1199
Colorado	12	989	Michigan	21	2313	Rhode Island	5	623
Connecticut	8	398	Minnesota	11	903	S. Carolina	7	583
Delaware	2	210	Mississippi	10	619	S. Dakota	7	607
Dist. of Columbia	7	355	Missouri	12	1760	Tennessee	11	778
Florida	27	2037	Montana	5	272	Texas	35	3557
Georgia	9	738	Nebraska	9	950	Utah	4	415
Hawaii	5	447	Nevada	4	281	Vermont	3	353
Idaho	3	280	New Hampshire	3	230	Virginia	12	1010
Illinois	55	3195	New Jersey	10	727	Washington	18	1980
Indiana	13	1162	New Mexico	8	953	West Virginia	5	504
Iowa	13	1422	New York	35	3697	Wisconsin	12	1290
Kansas	15	1832	N. Carolina	12	1041	Wyoming	4	238
			N. Dakota	5	416	TOTAL	634	60,663

Source: U.S. Department of Health and Human Services, 2003

Table 6.2. Child Care Arrangements Used by EHS Families

Percentage of children:	Full sample
Who received any child care	86%
Who received any center-based child care	51%

Percentage of children who received care in the following number of arrangements:	
0	14%
1	22%
2	25%
3	20%
4 or more	20%
Average number of arrangements used	2

Percentage of children who received care in more than one arrangement concurrently: 52%

Percentage of children whose primary child care arrangement was:	
Not in child care	14%
Early Head Start/Head Start	21%
Other child care center	17%
Nonrelative	14%
Parent or stepparent	8%
Grandparent or great-grandparent	18%
Other relative	8%

Percentage of children whose primary arrangement included care during:	
Evenings	30%
Early mornings	49%
Weekends	17%
Overnight	22%

Sample size: 920–988

Source: U.S. Department of Health and Human Services, Administration for Children and Families, 2002b

were enrolled in 2002 as part of the EHS expansion. Therefore, the totals reported in Table 6.1 reflect only those enrollees served in FY2002 prior to the EHS expansion.

EHS providers deliver services for pregnant women, infants, and toddlers through several different program approaches including center-based care, a home-based option in which families are supported through weekly home visits and group socialization experiences, locally designed program models, and accommodation option with a mix of center-based and home-based care.

EARLY HEAD START AND CHILD CARE

The majority of EHS children are in child care (see Table 6.2). EHS children across all program approaches use child care, and their use of child care increases as children get older. In one study of child care and Early Head Start, by 14 months of age, half of the EHS children received at least 30 hours of child care a week and by 36 months of age, two thirds of the EHS children were in care 30 or more hours a week. The study also showed that being in EHS increased the probability of children experiencing child care at every age — at 36 months, 84% of EHS children were in child care for at least 10 hours a week, compared to 78% of control children. At 14 months, 66% of EHS program children versus 57% of control group children were in 10 hours of child care or more. Some EHS children also needed child care during nonstandard work hours — at 24 months, 34% of all EHS children had received care in their primary arrangement during evening hours and 21% had received care during weekend hours (U.S. Department of Health and Human Services, Administration for Children and Families, 2003b).

It is important to note how being in EHS impacted the quality of child care that children were receiving, especially given that one of the goals of the Advisory Committee was for EHS children to receive good quality child care. The quality of child care was consistently good in EHS centers. Across all forms of center care, EHS children were three times more likely to be receiving their primary care in a good quality center than were control group children when they were 14 and 24 months old and almost one and one-half times more likely to be in good quality center care at 36 months (U.S. Department of Health and Human Services, Administration for Children and Families, 2003b). The quality of child care for EHS children was assessed when the children were 14, 24, and 36 months old (U.S. Department of Health and Human Services, Administration for Children and Families, 2003b). The study also found that at 28 months after program enrollment, 95% of EHS parents were satisfied with their primary child care arrangement.

PART C OF THE INDIVIDUALS WITH DISABILITIES EDUCATION ACT (IDEA): EARLY INTERVENTION FOR BABIES AND TODDLERS WITH DISABILITIES

Most babies develop and grow in predictable ways; they walk, talk, and gain new skills on schedule. For some young children, however, development unfolds according to a slower timetable or in an atypical fashion. The reason for a problem in early development may be physical, mental, environmental, or a combination of factors. Often the cause remains unknown and the future uncertain. What we do know, however, is that extremely premature babies, babies with genetic conditions such as Down syndrome, and young children with physical disabilities such as cerebral palsy or spina bifida, among others, need and respond to supportive interventions. Part C of the Individuals with Disabilities Education Act (IDEA) is the federal program that ensures that these children and their families are given the best chance for a productive and healthy start.

Part C authorizes the federal support for early intervention programs for babies and toddlers with disabilities, and provides federal assistance for states to maintain and implement statewide systems of services for eligible children, age birth through 2 years, and their families. Under Part C, all participating states and jurisdictions must provide early intervention services to any child below age 3 who is experiencing developmental delays or has a diagnosed physical or mental condition that has a high probability of resulting in a developmental delay. In addition, states may choose to provide services for babies and toddlers who are "at-risk" for serious developmental problems, defined as circumstances (including biological or environmental conditions or both) that will seriously affect the child's development unless interventions are provided. All states and territories are currently participating in the Part C program.

The incidence of babies and toddlers with disabilities is not clear. Estimates of children with disabilities range from 3% to 5.2% for children under age 3 to 8% to 14.1% for children under age 5 (March of Dimes, 2001; U.S. Department of Health and Human Services, 1995; Elinson, Kennedy & Verbrugge, 1998). Given these estimates, up to 5.5 million children under age 18 may have disabilities (8% of all children), including as many as 1.4 million children under age 3.

More male children age birth to 4 years have disabilities (4% of all children age birth to 17 years) than do girls of the same age (2.4%; Federal Interagency Forum on Child and Family Statistics, 2002).

Some disabilities seem to be on the rise. Autism and other conditions within the autism spectrum, for example, are now estimated to occur at a rate of 1 in 500 children (Filipek et al., 2000). The incidence of autism alone has increased over the last 10 years from 2 per 10,000 children to 3 to 4 per 1000 children (Yeargin-Allsopp et al., 2003). This means that of the 4 million babies born last year, 12,000 to 16,000 might be identified with autism or another disorder within the autism spectrum as they reach age 3.

While some disabilities are increasing dramatically, with no known cause for the increase, the incidence of other disabilities remain steady and some are decreasing. Reports of fetal alcohol syndrome, characterized by mental retardation, seizures, and behavior and learning problems caused by alcohol use during pregnancy, are less than half what they were 10 years ago. Table 6.3 shows the trend in incidence for some conditions with established developmental risk. Increases in autism, multiple births, and prematurity, as well as improved survival of very low birth-weight babies may be a factor in the rising number of children in need of specialized services and supports through Part C.

Families whose incomes are below 200% of poverty are almost 50% more likely to have a child with a disability than are families whose incomes are above 200% of poverty (Lee, Sills, & Oh, 2002). A national study of infants and toddlers in early intervention reports that there are more families on public assistance in the Part C system (42%) than in the general population (13%; Hebbeler et al., 2001).

Children in foster care are substantially overrepresented among those in early intervention (U.S. Department of Education, 2001). Of the babies and toddlers entering programs for children with disabilities and developmental delays, 7% were in foster care at the time of entry, about 10 times the rate of children in the general population who are in foster care (Hebbeler et al., 2001).

There are gaps in services to children with disabilities. Child care in particular is difficult to find for children with disabilities. In one multi-state study, 45% of mothers of an infant with a disability reported that they were not planning to work because they could not find child care, and 31% indicated that they could not find affordable child care (Booth & Kelly, 1998, 1999). In families whose children were enrolled in the Part C program, almost all of the fathers (90%) and nearly half of the mothers were employed; 22% of the mothers worked full-time (U.S. Department of Education, 2001).

According to *From Neurons to Neighborhoods*, "available evidence suggests that children with disabilities begin child care at older ages, are enrolled for fewer hours, are more likely to be cared for by relatives, and less likely to be in child care centers than other children" (Shonkoff & Phillips, 2000, p. 325).

The number of young children currently served by the Part C program has increased from a total of 165,351 in 1994 (the first year that state-reported data are considered reliable) to 247,433 in 2001. Table 6.4 shows growth in the Part C program, and Table 6.5 provides current state-by-state data.

EARLY HEAD START SERVICES FOR INFANTS AND TODDLERS WITH DELAYS OR DISABILITIES

Infants and toddlers in families with low incomes face a higher risk of delays and disabilities. Children in families with low incomes who receive early educational intervention starting in infancy have higher scores on mental, reading, and math tests than do children who don't receive the intervention (Oser & Cohen, 2003).

EHS is an active partner with community Part C early intervention systems for young children with disabilities. EHS provides an inclusive "natural environment" for children with disabilities. EHS also plays an active role in early identification of children with developmental delays or disabilities. In 2001–2002, 6,568 infants and toddlers in EHS were eligible for Part C early intervention, and 6,391 of these children actually received Part C services. This represents 10.5% of all EHS enrollees who received Part C early intervention services (U.S. Department of Health and Human Services, 2003).

Table 6.3. Incidence of Selected Birth Conditions With Established Developmental Risk (Rate per 100,000 Live Births), 1990–1999

Birth Condition	1990	1995	1999
Cleft lip/palate	77	80	79
Down syndrome	47	42	44
Fetal alcohol syndrome	13	7	4
Hydrocephalus	26	27	21
Microcephalus	9	8	6
Spina bifida	23	26	20

Source: Centers for Disease Control and Prevention, 2003a

Table 6.4. Infants and Toddlers With Disabilities Served in Part C, 1994–2001
(Includes 50 states and Outlying Areas) by Age and Percentage of Population

	1994	1995	1996	1997
Number served:				
Birth to age 1	29,617	29,790	31,496	34,375
Age 1 to 2 years	55,284	559,186	60,233	62,699
Age 2 to 3 years	80,450	88,310	94,798	99,263
Total children 0–3 served	165,351	177,286	186,527	196,337
Percentage of 0–3 population	1.56%	1.74%	1.75%	1.86%

	1998	1999	2000	2001
Number served:				
Birth to age 1	31,089	35,554	36,570	37,378
Age 1 to 2 years	60,558	66,373	74,260	78,396
Age 2 to 3 years	95,708	102,359	121,985	131,659
Total children 0–3 served	187,355	204,286	232,815	247,433
Percentage of 0–3 population	1.84%	1.87%	2.15%	not available

Source: U.S. Department of Education, Office of Special Education Programs, Data Analysis System, 2003

Table 6.5. Number of Infants and Toddlers Served in Part C (States and Outlying Areas), 2001

STATE	CHILD COUNT			
	AGE 0	AGE 1	AGE 2	AGE 0–2
Alabama	239	740	1,107	2,086
Alaska	90	195	339	624
Arizona	417	1,035	1,472	2,924
Arkansas	413	962	1,399	2,774
California	4,967	8,407	11,051	24,425
Colorado	696	1,307	2,041	4,044
Conneticut	442	1,094	2,343	3,879
Delaware	176	305	422	903
District Of Columbia	19	101	159	279
Florida	2,874	4,455	7,113	14,442
Georgia	485	1,151	1,876	3,512
Hawaii	1,919	995	1,047	3,961
Idaho	216	393	648	1,257
Illinois	998	3,365	5,658	10,021
Indiana	1,768	2,979	4,418	9,165
Iowa	241	508	888	1,637
Kansas	439	852	1,447	2,738
Kentucky	458	1,314	2,038	3,810
Louisiana	319	750	1,242	2,311
Maine	69	266	612	947
Maryland	563	1,479	2,858	4,900
Massachusetts	2,198	4,000	6,708	12,906
Michigan	1,226	2,346	3,522	7,094
Minnesota	388	871	1,793	3,052
Mississippi	336	660	1,034	2,030
Missouri	309	873	1,643	2,825

STATE	CHILD COUNT AGE 0	AGE 1	AGE 2	AGE 0–2
Montana	164	220	216	600
Nebraska	117	296	540	953
Nevada	116	306	473	895
New Hampshire	164	364	646	1,174
New Jersey	679	1,952	3,781	6,412
New Mexico	313	607	914	1,834
New York	2,313	7,854	20,250	30,417
North Carolina	711	2,054	2,890	5,655
North Dakota	63	142	166	371
Ohio	1,103	2,708	3,801	7,612
Oklahoma	577	899	1,151	2,627
Oregon	217	602	1,068	1,887
Pennsylvania	1,644	3,383	5,164	10,191
Rhode Island	177	309	602	1,088
South Carolina	289	695	1,109	2,093
South Dakota	82	201	372	655
Tennessee	820	1,590	2,291	4,701
Texas	2,767	5,918	9,486	18,171
Utah	433	820	1,241	2,494
Vermont	60	140	271	471
Virginia	550	1,688	2,505	4,743
Washington	340	1,038	1,741	3,119
West Virginia	315	540	698	1,553
Wisconsin	680	1,492	3,040	5,212
Wyoming	81	172	278	531
Guam	44	64	82	190
Northern Marianas	7	15	26	48
Puerto Rico	222	855	1,906	2,983
Virgin Islands	65	69	73	207
States Total:	**37,378**	**78,396**	**131,659**	**247,433**

Source: U.S. Department of Education, Office of Special Education Programs, Data Analysis System, 2003.

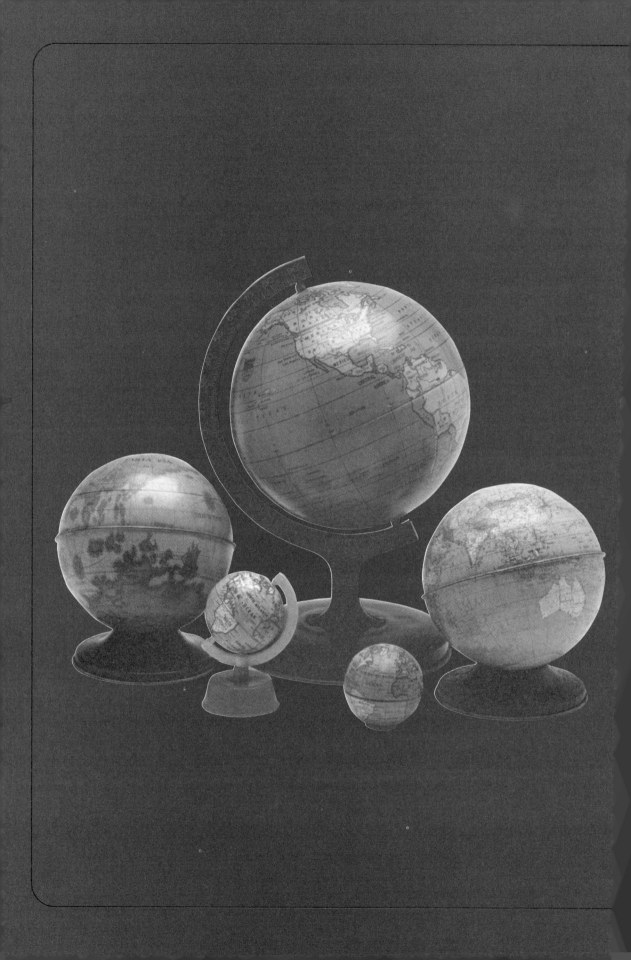

CHAPTER 7
INTERNATIONAL PERSPECTIVES

"Paradoxically, the world's greatest strength resides in its smallest citizens. From birth to age 3, the seeds of personhood — indeed, of nationhood — are taking root in every child. Synapses crackle and the patterns of a lifetime are established. In a remarkable 36 months, the brain develops, and children acquire the ability to think, speak, learn, and reason. This is the foundation for the values and social behavior of the adults they will one day become.

"These first 3 years of life offer an exceptional opportunity: Each time a child enters the world, there is the chance to break the relentless intergenerational cycles of poverty, violence and deprivation. By protecting the rights of this child and thousands of others and carefully nurturing them through the earliest stages of development, a nation can give a new generation the keys to unlocking the vast potential that may have been denied to the parents. For a government that wants to improve the lot of its people, investing in the first years of life is the best money it can spend. But tragically, both for children and for nations, these are the years that receive the least attention" (United Nations Children's Fund, 2002).

The first six chapters in this book presented data about America's babies. However, the issues addressed do not solely impact infants and toddlers in the United States. These issues — ranging from family economics, to immunizations, to early care and education — affect babies around the world. Mothers, fathers, policymakers, and advocates in other countries are concerned about many of the same issues and have addressed these issues in unique ways in their own countries. In this chapter, we provide a glimpse of some of these issues.

The United States is the third most populous country, with a population of 278,059,000.

—geographyIQ, 2003.

POPULATION TRENDS

The world's population is currently 6 billion people. China is the most populous country at 1,273,110,000 residents followed by India at 1,029,990,000. The United States is the third most populous country with a population of 278,059,000 (geographyIQ, 2003). Table 7.1 compares demographics for the United States, Canada, and Mexico.

Fertility rates are falling in virtually every country in the world except the United States and France. The United Nations projects that the world's population could "level off" at approximately nine billion by mid-century and then begin to decline (United Nations Population Division, 2003). Reasons for the decline in fertility rates include: improved education; greater employment opportunities and more financial independence for women; increased urbanization (making it harder to sustain more than one or two children; and increased availability of contraceptives (United Nations Population Division, 2003).

Globally, 57% of all babies are delivered by a health care professional such as a doctor, nurse, or midwife. In more developed countries, virtually all births (99%) are attended by a health care professional while in less-developed countries, 50% are attended by a skilled provider (Population Reference Bureau, 2002).

Life expectancy is one way to gauge the overall health of a country. Babies with the highest life expectancy in the world are Japanese girls. A baby girl born today in Japan can expect to live to be 84 years old (Population Reference Bureau, 2003a). The countries with highest life expectancy are listed in Table 7.2.

POVERTY

An analysis commissioned by the United Nations Children's Fund of the most recent data from the Luxembourg Study of household surveys indicates that the proportion of children living in poverty in 23 nations of the Organisation for Economic Co-operation and Development (OECD) varies from under 3% to more than 25%. The OECD has 29 members; these countries produce two thirds of the world's goods and services (United Nations Children's Fund, 2000). The Nordic countries – Denmark, Finland, Norway, and Sweden – have child poverty rates at around 5%. The United States comes in second to last (above Mexico) with the percentage of children living in relative poverty at 22.4% (see Table 7.3).

Table 7.1. Comparative Demographics, United States, Canada, and Mexico, 2001

	Population	Growth rate	Birth rate	Migration rate per 1000 population	Infant mortality rate deaths per 1000 live births	Life expectancy at birth (in years)
Canada	31,592,805	.99%	11.21/1000	6.13	5.02	79.56
Mexico	101,879,171	1.5%	22.77/1000	-2.77	25.36	71.76
United States	278,058,881	.9%	14.2/1000	3.5	6.76	77.26

Source: geographyIQ, 2003

Table 7.2. Life Expectancy at Birth, Top Ranked Countries, 1997

Female		Male	
Japan	84 years	Iceland	77 years
Switzerland	83	Japan	77
San Marino	83	Sweden	77
Australia	82	Australia	76
France	82	Canada	76
Iceland	82	Greece	76
Martinique	82	Norway	76
Spain	82	Switzerland	76
Sweden	82		
United States	80	United States	74

Source: Population Reference Bureau, 2003a

POVERTY IN LONE-PARENT FAMILIES

One factor that is related to child poverty in industrialized nations is the increase in the number of lone-parent families (United Nations Children's Fund, 2000). Lone-parent families are defined as families in which there is only one adult (and at least one child). A child living in a household with either one working adult or no working adult is more likely to fall below the poverty line than a child in a two-income house-hold (United Nations Children's Fund, 2000). Yet this does not mean that the greater the share of children living in lone-parent families, the higher the child poverty rate. For example, Sweden has a higher proportion of its children living in lone-parent fam-ilies than the United States or the United Kingdom and yet Sweden's child poverty rate is under 3% as compared to 22% and 19% in the United States and the United Kingdom respectively. Countries with the highest and lowest child poverty rates are listed in Table 7.4.

INFANT MORTALITY

Infant death rates vary considerably among countries. UNICEF uses a combined under-5 mortality rate (U5MR) as a critical indicator of the well-being of children. This represents the overall probability of dying between birth and 5 years of age (expressed as deaths per 1,000 live births). The countries with the highest and lowest U5MR are displayed in Table 7.5.

BREAST-FEEDING

Optimal breast-feeding practices include exclusive breast-feeding for the first 6 months of life. This goal is not being met. During the 1990s, modest improvements were made in exclusive breast-feeding; rates increased from 48% to 52% in the

Table 7.3 Child Poverty Rates (Households with income below 50% of the national median)

Countries with lowest child poverty

Sweden	2.6 %
Norway	3.9 %
Finland	4.3 %
Belgium	4.4 %
Luxembourg	4.5 %

Countries with highest child poverty

Mexico	26.2 %
United States	22.4 %
Italy	20.5 %
United Kingdom	19.8 %
Turkey	19.7 %

Table 7.4. Child Poverty in Lone-Parent Families

Countries With the Lowest Rates

	Poverty rate	% of all children in lone-parent families
Sweden	6.7 %	21.3 %
Finland	7.1 %	11.8 %
Hungary	10.4 %	7.4 %
Norway	13.1 %	15.0 %
Belgium	13.5 %	8.2 %

Countries With the Highest Rates

	Poverty rate	% of all children in lone-parent families
United States	55.4 %	16.6 %
Canada	51.6 %	12.2 %
Germany	51.2 %	9.8 %
Ireland	46.4 %	8.0 %
United Kingdom	45.6 %	20.0 %

Source: United Nations Children's Fund, 2000

Source: United Nations Children's Fund, 2000

developing world (United Nations Children's Fund, 2003a). Fewer than half of all infants are now being exclusively breast-fed for up to 4 months. As noted in Figure 7.1, the highest rates of exclusive breast-feeding are found in East Asia and the Pacific at 57% while the lowest are found in the former USSR/Baltic States region at 17%.

CHILD IMMUNIZATION

Timely immunization is a critical and cost-effective intervention that countries can provide to their young children. To be considered fully immunized, children must receive three doses of the DPT (diphtheria, pertussis, and tetanus) vaccine before their first birthday. The percentage of children receiving the third dose, DPT3, is an indicator of the extent to which routine immunization is provided. Global coverage with three doses of DPT vaccine increased from less than 38% in the beginning of the 1980s to 73% in 1990 (United Nations Children's Fund, 2003b). Figure 7.2 displays immunization coverage by region for 1999.

Vaccination programs are still underway to prevent poliovirus. The World Health Organization has a goal to eradicate polio by the year 2005. Tremendous progress has been made toward this goal. The number of countries still reporting polio cases has fallen from 120 in 1988 to 10 countries in 2002. Smallpox was eradicated in 1980 (Centers for Disease Control and Prevention, 2002b).

CHILD INJURY DEATHS

In some countries, the risk of a young child dying from an injury is still quite high. These rates vary from a high of 37 deaths per 100,000 children ages 1–4 in Korea, to a low of 5.6 deaths per 100,000 children in Sweden (see Table 7.6).

Table 7.5. Under-5 Mortality Rankings (U5MR), 2001

Highest

	U5MR value	Rank	Infant mortality rate
Sierra Leone	316	1	147 /1,000 births
Niger	265	2	124 /1,000 births
Angola	260	3	194 /1,000 births
Afghanistan	257	4	147/1,000 births
Liberia	235	5	132 /1,000 births

Lowest

	U5MR value	Rank	Infant mortality rate
Sweden	3	193	3.5 /1,000 births
Singapore	4	189	3.6 /1,000 births
Norway	4	189	3.9 /1,000 births
Iceland	4	189	3.6 /1,000 births
Denmark	4	189	5.0 /1,000 births
United States	8	158	6.8 /1,000 births

Source: United Nations Children's Fund, 2002; geographyIQ, 2003

Table 7.6. Injury Deaths in Children 1–4 years of age, 1991–1995 (deaths per 100,000 children)

Highest

Korea	37
Mexico	27.2
Portugal	23.8
New Zealand	19.6
United States	19.1

Lowest

Sweden	5.6
Italy	5.9
Finland	7.3
United Kingdom	7.3
Norway	8

Source: Clearinghouse on International Developments in Child, Youth and Family Policies, 2001a

Figure 7.1. Breast-feeding Rates by Region
(at 4 months of age), 1995–2000

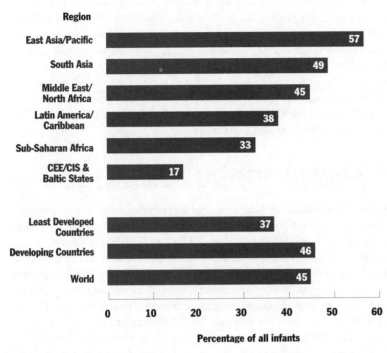

Source: United Nations Children Fund, 2003a

Figure 7.2. Immunization Coverage (DPT3) by Region, 1999

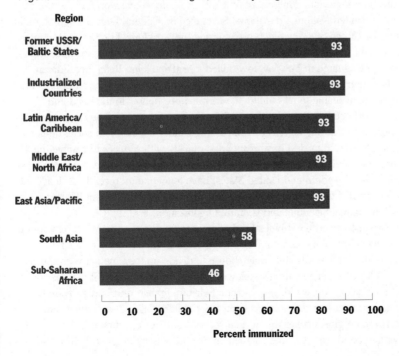

Source: United Nations Children's Fund, 2003b

PARENTAL LEAVE

Many countries provide mandatory job protection and paid maternity and/or parental leave policies for mothers and fathers in the labor force. The amount, duration, benefit level, and job protections vary. In contrast to Organisation for Economic Co-operation and Development (OECD) countries, the United States provides a brief parental leave time (12 weeks) without pay.

Across OECD countries, the average duration of parental leave is 44 weeks (10 months), with paid leave lasting an average of 36 weeks (Clearinghouse on International Developments in Child, Youth and Family Policies, 2001b). Table 7.7 notes parental leave policies in OECD countries.

EARLY CARE AND EDUCATION

Early care and education for very young children is an issue that many countries are grappling with, both in terms of meeting the demand and ensuring quality services. Demographic changes are creating the demand for early childhood services. These changes include rapid urbanization, the movement of men and women from agricultural to non-agricultural work, and the need for a highly educated, competitive workforce (United Nations Educational Scientific and Cultural Organization, 2002a). For example, a recent study reported that as parents moved from informal to formal work settings, they were not at home to care for the children or the workplace was unsafe so that their children could no longer accompany them to work. Children 5 years old and younger were left home alone or in the care of young school age children when families lacked access to child care. Extended family members are not filling the child care gap — urbanization separates parents from extended family, and adult members of the extended families are often working or caring for others, especially in countries with high rates of HIV/AIDS. The report concluded that access to child care is an important component of assuring a competitive workforce in the global economy (United Nations Educational Scientific and Cultural Organization, 2002a).

As in the United States, women are entering the workforce in other countries at higher rates than ever before. Women are now 40% of the global workforce; they continue to be situated in low-pay, low-skilled jobs (Population Reference Bureau, 2002). In countries other than the United States, child care is seen as a public service that should be available to all families. Government responses to the need and demand of early childhood education and family benefits in developed countries vary. Those with a strong conviction concerning gender equality and social democracy (e.g., the Nordic countries) have responded quickly with services to resolve the needs of family and work while countries with liberal and market-oriented ideologies (e.g., the United Kingdom and United States) have tended, until recently, to leave the matter up to individual families with minimal government involvement (United Nations Educational Scientific and Cultural Organization, 2002b).

The Swedish government helps fund parents to take care of their own children by paying 80% of a parent's salary for up to 1 year after the birth of a child. This applies to either parent and they may choose to divide up the time between the two of them (Polk, 1997). They are also allowed to take up to 60 days off per year at 80% of their salary to care for a sick child. Belgium, France, and Italy provide high quality universal care in state-run preschools for children ages 3–6 (Kamerman, 2000). These programs cover the normal school day (7 or 8 hours a day) and also have "wrap-around" services that supplement the school day program before and

Table 7.7. Maternity/Paternity Leave in Organisation for Economic
Co-operation and Development Countries, 1995–1996

Country	Duration in weeks	Benefit % of wage	Other paternity leave
Australia	52	unpaid	—
Austria	16	100	Parental leave, 2 years at partial wage
Belgium	15	75-80	Paternity, 3 days; Parental, 6 months
Canada	17	15 weeks at 55, 2 unpaid	Parental, 10 weeks at 55%
Czech Republic	28	69	—
Denmark	28	100	Paternity, 2 weeks; Parental, 12 months at 90% of UIB* rate
Finland	18	70	Paternity, 2 weeks; Parental, 26 weeks at 70%
France	16	100	Paternity, 3 days; Parental leave with 2 or more children, 3 years flat rate
Germany	14	100	Parental leave until child is 3; 2 years flat rate, 1 year unpaid
Greece	16	50	—
Hungary	24	100	Income-tested child-rearing rate
Iceland	24	80	3 months for each parent, unpaid
Ireland	14	70	—
Italy	20	80	Parental leave, 6 months at 30%
Japan	14	60	6 weeks prenatal, 8 weeks post-birth
Korea-South	no statutory leave		
Luxembourg	16	100	—
Mexico	12	100	—
Netherlands	16	100	Unemployed mothers at lower rate; parental leave, 6 months per parent part-time, unpaid
New Zealand	14	unpaid	2 weeks paternity; 52 weeks parental, including 14 weeks maternity
Norway	52	80	or 42 weeks at 100%; paternity leave 4 weeks; child rearing leave up to age 2
Poland	16/18/26	100	16 weeks for first child, 18 for subsequent, 26 for multiple births; additional 24 months (36 for single parent) at flat rate.
Portugal	24	100	Up to 24 months unpaid parental leave
Spain	16	100	2 days paternity at 100%; unpaid parental leave up to age 3
Sweden	52	80	60 days prior to delivery; additional 3 months at flat rate plus 3 months unpaid up to 8 years; 6 months extra for each child of multiple birth
Switzerland	16	varies	—
Turkey	12	66 2/3	—
United Kingdom	18	6 wks at 90; 12 weeks at low flat rate	13 weeks unpaid up to child's 5th birthday
United States	12	unpaid	—

* UIB = unemployment insurance benefits

Source: Clearinghouse on International Developments in Child, Youth, and Family Policies, 2000

after school, at lunchtime, and during school holidays at income-related fees (Kamerman, 2000).

In some countries, up to 97% of all children between the ages of 3 and 6 years are in early childhood education and care (see Table 7.8). For infants and toddlers (age birth to 3 years), Denmark reports the highest enrollment, at 58% of all children over age 1 enrolled in early education and care.

LITERACY WORLDWIDE

In the United States and other industrialized countries, the adult literacy rate is 97% overall (98% of men and 96% of women). In less economically developed countries, the rates are 79% for men and 62% for women while in the least developed countries literacy rates are 60% for men and 38% for women (Population Reference Bureau, 2003c). In most societies, being more educated also means being wealthier; educational attainment is often used as a proxy for economic status. This may partially explain why there is such a strong correlation between level of maternal education and infant survival rates. On average, for every year of additional schooling a girl receives, her chance of having a baby die is reduced by 10% and her expected income rises by 10%–20% (Population Reference Bureau, 2003c).

Table 7.8. Children in Early Childhood Education and Care (as a percentage of all children)

Country	Percentage of all children	
	Age birth–3 years	Age 3–6 years
Australia	—	80
Austria	3	80
Belgium	30	97
Denmark	58*	83
Finland	48*	73
France	29	99
Germany	5	85
Ireland	2	55
Italy	6	95
Japan	21	52
Luxembourg	N/A	N/A
Netherlands	8	71
New Zealand	25	85
Norway	N/A	N/A
Portugal	12	48
Spain	5	84
Sweden	48*	79
United Kingdom	2	60**
United States	26	71

* From age 1, when basic paid leave ends; all three countries have supplementary paid and job protected parental or child rearing leaves.
** 3- and 4-year-olds only, because compulsory school begins at age 5.
Source: Kamerman, 2000.

APPENDIX A. DATA SOURCES

Except for the AFCARS description, all data source information was compiled by Tim Champney, Ph.D., Delmarva Foundation for Medical Care.

Adoption and Foster Care Analysis and Reporting System (AFCARS)

The Adoption and Foster Care Analysis and Reporting System (AFCARS) is a federally mandated data collection system designed to collect case level information on all children covered by the protections of Title IV-B/E of the Social Security Act (Section 427). States are required to collect data on all children in foster care for whom the state child welfare agency has responsibility for placement, care, or supervision and on children who are adopted under the auspices of the State's public child welfare agency. States are required to submit AFCARS data semi-annually to the Administration for Children and Families. http://www.acf.hhs.gov/programs/cb/dis/afcars

Current Population Survey

Core survey and supplements. The Current Population Survey (CPS) is a monthly nationwide survey of about 50,000 households conducted for the Bureau of Labor Statistics by the U.S. Census Bureau. At present, there are 754 CPS sampling areas in the United States, with coverage in every State and the District of Columbia.

Information about the CPS is available online at http://www.bls.census.gov/cps/cpsmain.htm.

National Health Interview Survey

The National Health Interview Survey (NHIS) is a continuing nationwide sample survey of the noninstitutionalized civilian population in which data are collected during personal household interviews.

The NHIS sample includes an oversample of black and Hispanic persons and is designed to allow the development of national estimates of health conditions, health service utilization, and health problems of the noninstitutionalized civilian population of the United States. The response rate for the ongoing part of the survey has been between 94% and 98% over the years. In 1997, the NHIS was redesigned; estimates beginning in 1997 are likely to vary slightly from those for previous years.

Interviewers collected information for the basic questionnaire on 100,618 persons in 2000, including 28,495 children.

Information about the NHIS is available online at http://www.cdc.gov/nchs/nhis.htm.

National Immunization Survey

The National Immunization Survey (NIS) is a continuing nationwide telephone sample survey of families with children ages 19–35 months. Estimates of vaccine-specific coverage are available for the nation, the states, and 28 urban areas.

Information about the NIS is available online at http://www.nisabt.org and on the NIS website at http://www.cdc.gov/NIP/coverage.

National Linked File of Live Births and Infant Deaths

The National Linked File of Live Births and Infant Deaths is a data file for research on infant mortality. Beginning with the 1995 data, this file is produced in two formats. National linked files are available starting with the birth cohort of 1983. No linked file was produced for the 1992 through 1994 data years. Match completeness for each of the birth cohort files is about 98%.

Information about the National Linked File of Live Births and Infant Deaths is available online at http://www.cdc.gov/nchs/linked.htm.

National Vital Statistics System

Through the National Vital Statistics System, the National Center for Health Statistics (NCHS) collects and publishes data on births and deaths in the United States. NCHS obtains information on births and deaths from the registration offices of all states, New York City, and the District of Columbia.

Demographic information on birth certificates, such as race and ethnicity, is provided by the mother at the time of birth. Hospital records provide the base for information on prenatal care, while funeral directors and family members provide demographic information on death certificates. Medical certification of cause of death is provided by a physician, medical examiner, or coroner.

Information about the National Vital Statistics System is available online at http://www.cdc.gov/nchs/nvss.htm.

Population Projections

National population projections begin with recent population estimates by age, race, and Hispanic origin. These statistics are then projected forward to 2050, based on assumptions about fertility, mortality, and international migration. Low, middle, and high growth assumptions are made for each of these components. The current middle series assumptions are that:

• Fertility will see little change over time, with levels for each race/ethnic group converging to about 2.1 children per woman in the long run.

• Mortality will continue to improve, with life expectancy for each race/ethnic group converging to about 90 years by 2100.

• Net international migration will decline somewhat in the near term but increase after 2010, with a relatively larger portion from Asia and Africa and a relatively smaller portion from Latin America.

For more information, see U.S. Bureau of the Census. (1996). *Population projections of the United States by age, sex, race, and Hispanic origin* (1130, Series P25). Washington, DC: U.S. Bureau of the Census.

Information about population projections is available online at http://www.census.gov/population/www/projections/popproj.html.

Survey of Income and Program Participation

Core survey and topical modules. Implemented by the U.S. Census Bureau since 1984, the Survey of Income and Program Participation (SIPP) is a continuous series of national longitudinal panels, with a sample size ranging from approximately 14,000 to 36,700 interviewed households. The duration of each panel ranges from 2 1/2 years to 4 years, with household interviews every 4 months.

The SIPP collects detailed information on income, labor force participation, participation in government assistance programs, and general demographic characteristics to measure the effectiveness of existing government programs, to estimate future costs and coverage of government programs, and to provide statistics on the distribution of income in America. In addition, topical modules provide detailed information on a variety of subjects, including health insurance, child care, adult and child well-being, marital and fertility history, and education and training.

Information about the SIPP is available online at http://www.sipp.census.gov/sipp.

National Summary of Injury Mortality Data

The Injury Mortality Data available on the CDC World Wide Web pages provide tabulations of the total numbers of deaths and the death rates per 100,000 population for major and other selected external causes of death from injury, by race, sex, and age groupings. National data on injury mortality are from 1979 through 1997 and allows users to assess short-term trends in numbers of deaths and death rates. State figures summarize national and state data for 1989 through 1997 for selected causes of injury mortality.

Note: in previous versions of these web pages, a different source of population estimates were used for the years 1991–1995. This change may result in some different rates between the current and previous rates presented for 1991–1995 only.

Centers for Disease Control and Prevention National Center for Health Statistics

Through the National Vital Statistics System, the National Center for Health Statistics (NCHS) collects and publishes data on births, deaths, marriages, and divorces in the United States. In most areas practically all births and deaths are registered. The most recent test of the completeness of birth registration, conducted on a sample of births from 1964 to 1968, showed that 99.3% of all births in the United States during that period were registered. No comparable information is available for deaths, but it is generally believed that death registration in the United States is at least as complete as birth registration.

Birth File

The birth file is comprised of demographic and medical information from birth certificates. Demographic information, such as race and ethnicity, is provided by the mother at the time of birth. Medical and health information is based on hospital records. Additional information follows for selected items on the birth certificate.

Race–Data on birth rates, birth characteristics, and fetal death rates for 1980 and more recent years for liveborn infants and fetal deaths are presented in this report according to race of mother, unless specified otherwise. Before 1980 data were tabulated by race of newborn and fetus, taking into account the race of both parents. If the parents were of different races and one parent was white, the child was classified according to the race of the other parent. When neither parent was white, the child was classified according to father's race, with one exception: if either parent was Hawaiian, the child was classified Hawaiian. Before 1964, if race was unknown, the birth was classified as white. Beginning in 1964 unknown race was classified according to information on the previous record.

Maternal age–Mother's age was reported on the birth certificate by all states. Data are presented for mother's age 10–49 years through 1996 and 10–54 years starting in 1997, on the basis of the mother's date of birth or age as reported on the birth certificate. The age of mother is edited for upper and lower limits. When the age of the mother is computed to be under 10 years or 55 years or over (50 years or over in 1964–1996), it is considered not stated and imputed according to the age of the mother from the previous birth record of the same race and total birth order (total of fetal deaths and live births). Before 1963 not stated ages were distributed in proportion to the known ages for each racial group. Beginning in 1997 the birth rate for the maternal age group 45–49 years includes data for mother's age 50–54 years in the numerator and is based on the population of women 45–49 years in the denominator.

Maternal education–Mother's education was reported on the birth certificate by 38 states in 1970. Data were not available from Alabama, Arkansas, California, Connecticut,

Delaware, District of Columbia, Georgia, Idaho, Maryland, New Mexico, Pennsylvania, Texas, and Washington. Starting in 1992 mother's education was reported by all 50 states and the District of Columbia.

Marital status—Mother's marital status was reported on the birth certificate by 39 states and the District of Columbia in 1970, and by 38 States and the District of Columbia in 1975. The incidence of births to unmarried women in states with no direct question on marital status was assumed to be the same as the incidence in reporting states in the same geographic division. In 1998, all but two states (Michigan and New York) included a direct question about mother's marital status on their birth certificates.

Hispanic origin—Between 1983 and 1987, information on births of Hispanic parentage was available for 23 states and the District of Columbia. In 1990, 99% of birth records included information on mother's origin.

Tobacco use—Information on tobacco use during pregnancy became available for the first time in 1989 with revision of the U.S. Standard Birth Certificate. In 1989 data on tobacco use were collected by 43 states and the District of Columbia. During 1989–2000, California did not require the reporting of tobacco use in the standard format on the birth certificate.

Mortality File

The mortality data file is comprised of demographic and medical information from death certificates. Demographic information is provided by the funeral director based on information supplied by an informant. Medical certification of cause of death is provided by a physician, medical examiner, or coroner. The mortality data file is a fundamental source of cause-of-death information by demographic characteristics and for geographic areas, such as states. The mortality file is one of the few sources of comparable health-related data for smaller geographic areas in the United States and over a long time period. Mortality data can be used not only to present the characteristics of those dying in the United States, but also to determine life expectancy and to compare mortality trends with other countries.

Infant and maternal mortality rates are calculated with denominators comprising the number of live births rather than population estimates. Starting with 1980, infant and maternal mortality trends are based on maternal race and ethnicity of the live birth in the denominator. Before 1980, infant and maternal mortality trends were based on child's race in the denominator, which took into account the race of both parents. Infant and maternal mortality trends for Hispanics began with 1985 and are based on Hispanic origin of mother.

Mortality data in *Health, United States* are presented for four major race groups, white, black, American Indian or Alaska Native, and Asian or Pacific Islander, in accordance with 1977 U.S. Office of Management and Budget (OMB) standards for presenting federal statistics on race. Over the next several years, major changes will occur in the way federal agencies collect and tabulate data on race and Hispanic origin, in accordance with the 1997 guidelines from OMB (see Appendix II, Race). The major difference between the 1977 and 1997 guidelines is adoption of data-collection procedures in which respondents can identify with more than one race group.

For more information, see: National Center for Health Statistics, Technical Appendix, *Vital Statistics of the United States, 2000, Vol. I,* Natality, and Vol. II, Mortality, Part A available on the NCHS home page at www.cdc.gov/nchs. Click on Vital Statistics, Birth Data and Mortality Data.

Population Bureau of the Census

The census of population has been taken in the United States every 10 years since 1790. In the 1990 and 2000 censuses, data were collected on sex, race, age, and marital status from 100% of the enumerated population. More detailed information such as income, education, housing, occupation, and industry were collected from a representative sample of the population. For most of the country, one out of six households (about 17%) received the more detailed questionnaire. In places of residence estimated to have less than 2,500 population, 50 percent of households received the long form. The question on race for Census 2000 was different from the one for the 1990 census in several ways. Most significantly, respondents were given the option of selecting one or more race categories to indicate their racial identities, For more information, see: U.S. Bureau of the Census, *1990 Census of Population, General Population Characteristics*, Series 1990, CP–1; or visit the Census Bureau home page at www.census.gov.

APPENDIX B: GLOSSARY

AFDC (Aid to Families with Dependent Children; Title IV A of the Social Security Act): AFDC, now replaced by TANF, was a means-tested public assistance program that provided financial aid for needy children and their caretakers.

Block Grants: Federal funds given to state or local government which must be spent for a general purpose specified by the grant. Block grants do not require preapproval for individual projects or programs as long as they are spent in the agreed upon area, such as some aspects of health, education, personal social services, and public assistance.

Child Care and Development Fund (CCDF): The Personal Responsibility and Work Opportunity Act of 1996 revamped the structure of federal funding for child care and created the CCDF. This streamlined block grant attempts to maximize states' flexibility in administering child care programs and establishes a single set of rules and regulations that apply to all components of the fund. CCDF funding is divided into three streams of federal funds: federal mandatory funds that do not require a state match, federal mandatory funds that do require a state match, and federal discretionary funds that do not require a state match.

Child Care Services: Out-of-home care of children under compulsory school age, or of primary school age children when school is not open. Includes preschool, pre-kindergarten, kindergarten, center-based care, family day care homes, and before and after school services.

Child Poverty Rate: Percentage of children living in families with incomes below the poverty threshold.

Child Welfare: Social policies for troubled children and their families that may include: child protective services, foster care, adoption, family preservation, residential treatment, and home or community-based services.

Discretionary Funding: Funding appropriated by Congress each year for a specific purpose.

Discretionary Programs: Social programs for which funding is appropriated each year.

Early Periodic Screening, Diagnosis, and Treatment (EPSDT): EPSDT is Medicaid's comprehensive and preventive child health program for individuals up to age 21. It was defined by law as part of the Omnibus Budget Reconciliation Act of 1989 (OBRA 89) legislation and includes periodic screening, vision, dental, and hearing services.

Earned Income Tax Credit: A refundable tax credit that allows low-income working parents to receive a credit against their income tax or a cash supplement if their taxable income falls below a certain amount.

Entitlement Program: A program that provides money or services to qualified beneficiaries as a legal right, based solely upon the specific status of the client (i.e., food stamps).

Family and Medical Leave Act (FMLA): FMLA requires public agencies and businesses with more than 50 employees to offer unpaid family leave of up to 12 weeks to parents of newborns, those who are adopting children, and those who must care for an ill family member.

Food Stamps: A 1964 federal program mandated nationally in 1974 providing vouchers for the purchase of food only. It is a means-tested program available to all individuals and families regardless of marital status or presence or absence of children who meet income and asset, employment, and other eligibility criteria.

Galactosemia: A condition resulting from a deficiency of an enzyme needed to metabolize milk sugar. Usually fatal unless treated with special milk-free infant formula.

Head Start/Early Head Start: A federally funded program for disadvantaged children and their parents (pregnant women, babies, toddlers, and preschoolers), designed to compensate for developmental and educational lags caused by social deprivation. Program approaches for delivering services in Early Head Start include: center-based programs, home-based programs, and mixed-approach programs.

Hypothyroidism: Congenital hypothyroidism is a condition, present at birth, in which the thyroid gland is either absent, or not producing enough thyroid hormones to ensure proper growth. Without treatment beginning shortly after birth and continuing for life, hypothyroidism results in mental retardation and limited physical development.

Immunization: The process by which a person becomes protected against a disease. This term is often used interchangeably with vaccination or inoculation.

Infant Mortality Rate (IMR) also called "Infant Death Rate": Annual deaths of babies under 1 year of age per 1,000 live births. More specifically, this is the probability of dying between birth and 1 year of age.

In-Kind Benefit: Noncash benefit in the form of a voucher, commodity, or service (i.e., food stamps, Section 8 housing vouchers, Medicaid, school meals, child care services, public education).

Low Birth Weight: Babies weighing less than 2,500 grams or 5 pounds 8 ounces. The lower an infant's birth weight below 2,500 grams, the greater the infant's vulnerability to infections and other problems and the greater the risk of sickness and death.

Medicaid (Title XIX of the Social Security Act): A means-tested program that pays for medical costs of categorical assistance recipients and specified other groups among the poor. Funded by federal and state (and sometimes local) government.

Multiple Births: The process by which more than one offspring is produced.

Part C of the Individuals with Disabilities Education Act (IDEA): Part C of the Individuals with Disabilities Education Act (IDEA) authorizes the creation of early intervention programs for babies and toddlers with disabilities, and provides federal assistance for states to maintain and implement statewide systems of services for eligible children, ages birth through 2 years, and their families. States and jurisdictions participating in Part C must provide early intervention services to any child below age 3 who is experiencing developmental delays, has a diagnosed physical or mental condition that has a high probability of resulting in a developmental delay, and some states serve children who are at-risk for serious developmental problems.

The Personal Responsibility and Work Opportunity Act of 1996: The new "welfare" law: replaces AFDC with TANF, sets time limits for receipt, mandates work, ends entitlement to assistance and provides block grant funding giving states great flexibility in designing the TANF program.

PKU (Phenylketonuria): a condition in which the body lacks the enzyme needed to process nutrients. Without the enzyme, phenylalanine accumulates in the cells, resulting in brain damage, mental retardation or learning disabilities, and behavior problems. Treated with a special, lifelong diet of phenylalanine-free foods including a special infant formula.

Prematurity: A newborn with a gestational age of less than 37 weeks. Traditionally, the definition of prematurity was a birth weight of less than 2500 grams, regardless of gestational age.

Preschool: Child care services to children below the age of formal public education that includes educational and developmental content.

Public Assistance: Cash benefit provided to the poor on the basis of a means test. Financed out of general tax revenues. Eligibility requirements and dollar amounts vary among states.

State Child Health Insurance Program (SCHIP): SCHIP gives states the option of expanding health coverage to children in families with incomes up to or above 200% of the poverty level.

Stillbirth: A baby born at 20 weeks gestation or later, who shows no sign of life.

Supply Subsidy: Direct funding to provider so that services are available to the client in the community (i.e., public health, housing, and child care).

Tax Benefits: Policy instruments that may act as income transfers for individuals or families. Two major categories: 1) allowances—pre-tax deductions (i.e., dependent or personal exemption); 2) credits—deductions taken against tax liability (i.e., child care tax credit); may be cash rebate when income is below tax threshold as in Earned Income Tax Credit.

Temporary Assistance to Needy Families (TANF): The new means-tested cash assistance program, replacing AFDC. Highlights of the program include: benefit levels vary by state, requires beneficiaries to go to work within 2 years of claiming the benefit, limits receipt to a maximum of 5 years overall, and funding is in the form of block grants to states giving states great flexibility in program design.

Very Low Birthweight: Babies weighing less than 1,500 grams or 3 pounds 4 ounces.

Vouchers: Form of demand subsidy (e.g., food stamps, Medicaid) which functions as a cash equivalent for the purchase of specified goods/services. They provide more freedom of choice than a specific service but less than a cash benefit.

Supplemental Food Program for Women, Infants and Children (WIC): Vouchers issued by the U.S. Department of Agriculture to provide for nutritional needs of low-income women, infants, and young children.

REFERENCES

American Academy of Pediatrics. (2000a). Changing concepts of sudden infant death syndrome: Implications for infants sleeping environment and sleep position. *Pediatrics, 105*(3), 650–656.

American Academy of Pediatrics, Committee on Early Childhood, Adoption, and Dependent Care. (2000b). Developmental issues for young children in foster care (Policy Statement). *Pediatrics, 106*(5), 1145–1150.

American Academy of Pediatrics. (2003). Positioning and SIDS: Update. Retrieved April 21, 2003, from www.aap.org/new/sids

American Academy of Pediatrics, Committee on Early Childhood, Adoption, and Dependent Care. (2002). Health care of young children in foster care (Policy Statement), *Pediatrics, 109*(3), 536–541.

American Academy of Pediatrics, Work Group on Breastfeeding. (1997). Breastfeeding and the use of human milk. *Pediatrics, 100*(6), 1035–1039.

American Association for Single People. (2003). 2000 census – AASP Report. Retrieved March 15, 2003, from www.singlesrights.com/Census%202000

American Association of Retired Persons. (2003). Grandparents raising grandchildren. Retrieved February 19, 2003, from www.aarp.org/confacts

American SIDS Institute. (n.d.) Sudden infant death syndrome: U.S. annual SIDS rate 1980–1998. Retrieved April 18, 2003, from www.sids.org

American Society for Reproductive Medicine. (1999, November). Guidelines on number of embryos transferred. Retrieved February 20, 2003, from www.asrm.org

American Society for Reproductive Medicine (2003a). Challenges of parenting multiples. Retrieved February 20, 2003, from www.asrm.org

American Society for Reproductive Medicine. (2003b). Fact sheet: In vitro fertilization. Retrieved April 21, 2003, from www.asrm.org

American Society for Reproductive Medicine. (2003c). Frequently asked questions about infertility. Retrieved April 21, 2003, from www.asrm.org

Arias, E. (2002). United States life tables, 2000. *National vital statistics report, 51*(3). Hyattsville, MD: National Center for Health Statistics.

Ayoub, C., Pan, B., Guinee, K., & Russell, C. (2001, April). *Relationships between family characteristics and young children's language and socio-emotional development families eligible for Early Head Start.* Paper presented at the Biennial Meeting of the Society for Research in Child Development, Minneapolis, MN.

Bachu, A., & O'Connell, M. (2000). Fertility of American women: June 1998. *Current Population Reports.* P20–526. Washington, DC: U.S. Census Bureau.

Barlow, S., and Dietz, W. (1998). Obesity evaluation and treatment: Expert committee recommendations. *Pediatrics, 102*, E29.

Barr, R. (1990) The normal crying curve: What do we know? *Developmental Medicine and Child Neurology, 32*, 356–362.

Beers, M., & Berkow, R. (1999). *The Merck manual of diagnosis and therapy.* Whitehouse Station, NJ: Merck Research Laboratories.

Beral, V., et al. (2002). Breast cancer and breastfeeding: Collaborative reanalysis of individual data from 47 epidemiological studies in 30 countries, including 50302 women with breast cancer and 96973 women without the disease. *The Lancet, 360* (9328), 187–195

Booth, C. L., & Kelly, J. F. (1998). Child care characteristics of infants with and without special needs: Comparisons and concerns. *Early Childhood Research Quarterly, 13,* 603–622.

Booth, C. L., & Kelly, J. F. (1999). Child care and employment in relation to infants' disabilities and risk factors. *American Journal on Mental Retardation, 104*(2), 117–130.

Brenner, R., Overpeck, M., Trumble, A., DerSimonian, R., & Berendes, H. (1999). Deaths attributable to injuries in infants, United States, 1983–1991. *Pediatrics, 103*(5), 968–974.

Bureau of Labor Statistics. (2003). Distribution of families by type and labor force status of family members, 1940–2000. Washington, DC: Current Population Survey.

Carter, L., & Stevens, C. (1999). Domestic violence and children. *The Future of Children, 1*(3), 2.

Centers for Disease Control and Prevention. (1995). Trends in length of stay for hospital deliveries – United States, 1970–1992. *Morbidity and Mortality Weekly Report, 44*(17), 335–337.

Centers for Disease Control and Prevention. (1998a). Assessment of infant sleeping position – selected states, 1996. *Morbidity and Mortality Weekly Report, 47*(41) 873–877.

Centers for Disease Control and Prevention. (1998b). *Pediatric nutrition surveillance: 1997 full report.* Atlanta, GA: U.S. Department of Health and Human Services.

Centers for Disease Control and Prevention. (2001a). *National immunization survey 2001.* Atlanta, GA: Author.

Centers for Disease Control and Prevention. (2001b). State-specific prevalence of current cigarette smoking among adults, and policies and attitudes about secondhand smoke – U.S. 2000. *Morbidity and Mortality Week Report, 50*(49), 1101–1106.

Centers for Disease Control and Prevention. (2002a). Longer hospital stays for childbirth. Retrieved April 23, 2003, from www.cdc.gov/nchs

Centers for Disease Control and Prevention. (2002b). Background on global polio eradication initiative. Retrieved March 14, 2003, from www.cdc.gov/nip/global/stopteam/backgrd.htm

Centers for Disease Control and Prevention. (2002c). Program in brief: Early hearing detection and intervention. Retrieved April 11, 2003, from www.cdc.gov/programs

Centers for Disease Control and Prevention. (2003a). Birth anomaly rate. Retrived March 18, 2003, from www.cdc.gov/nchs/about/major/natality/natdesc.htm

Centers for Disease Control and Prevention. (2003b). *Data 2010 healthy people 2010 database.* Retrieved March 29, 2003, from www.cdc.gov

Charney, E., Goodman, H. C., McBride, M., Lyon, B., and Pratt, R. (1976). Childhood antecedents of adult obesity: Do chubby infants become obese adults? *The New England Journal of Medicine, 295,* 6–9.

Child Trends. (2002). *Charting parenthood: A statistical portrait of fathers and mothers in America.* Washington, DC: Author.

Clearinghouse on International Developments in Child, Youth and Family Policies. (2000). Maternity and parental leaves, 1997–1999. Retrieved June 2, 2003, from www.childpolicyintl.org/familyleavetables/table111.pdf

Clearinghouse on International Developments in Child, Youth and Family Policies. (2001a). Injury deaths by age, 1991–1995. Retrieved April 28, 2003, from www.childpolicyintl.org/sihealth/table315.pdf

Clearinghouse on International Developments in Child, Youth and Family Policies. (2001b). New 12-country study reveals substantial gaps in U.S. early childhood education and care policies. Issue Brief, Summer. Retrieved May 30, 2003, from www.childpolicyintl.org/issuebrief/issuebrief1.htm

Colpe, L. (2000). Estimates of mental and emotional problems, functional impairments, and associated disability outcomes for the U.S. child population in households. Retrieved April 24, 2003, from www.mentalhealth.org/publications

Conners G., Veenema, T., Kavanaugh, C., Ricci, J., & Callahan, C. (2002). Still falling: A community wide infant walker injury prevention initiative. *Patient Education and Counseling, 46*(3), 169–173.

Consumer Product Safety Commission. (2000). Nursery products report. Retrieved March 11, 2003, from www.cpsc.gov/library/nursry00.pdf

Cost, Quality & Child Outcomes Study Team. (1995). *Cost, quality and child outcomes in child care centers: Executive summary* (2nd ed). Denver, CO: Economics Department, University of Colorado at Denver.

Davis, B., Moon, R., Sachs, H., & Ottolini, M. (1998). Effects of sleep position on infant motor development. *Pediatrics, 102*(5), 1135–1140.

Dicker, S., & Gordon, E. (2000). Connecting healthy development and permanency: A pivotal role for child welfare professionals. *Permanency Planning Today, 1*(1) 12–15.

Dicker, S., Gordon, E., & Knitzer, J. (2001). *Improving the odds for the healthy development of young children in foster care.* New York: National Center for Children in Poverty.

Dybing, E., & Sanner, T. (1999). Passive smoking, sudden infant death syndrome (SIDS) and childhood infections. *Human and Experimental Toxicology, 18,* 202–205.

DYG, Inc., Civitas, ZERO TO THREE, & Brio (2000). What grown-ups understand about child development: A national benchmark survey. Chicago: Author.

Ehrle, J., Adams, G., & Tout, T. (2001). *Who's caring for our youngest children: Child care patterns of infants and toddlers.* Washington, DC: The Urban Institute.

Elinson, L., Kennedy, G., & Verbrugge, L. (1998) Considering children with disabilities and the state children's health insurance program. Washington, DC: Office of Disability, Aging, and Long-Term Care Policy, U.S. Department of Health and Human Services.

Fantuzzo, J., & Mohr, W. (1999). Prevalence and effects of child exposure to domestic violence. *The future of children: Domestic violence and children, 9*(3), 21–32.

Federal Interagency Forum on Child and Family Statistics. (2002). *America's children: Key national indicators of child well-being, 2002.* Washington, DC: U.S. Government Printing Office.

Fields, J., & Casper, L. (2001). America's families and living arrangements: Population characteristics. *Current Population Reports.* Washington, DC: U.S. Census Bureau.

Filipek, P.A., et al. (2000). Practice parameters: Screening and diagnosis of autism: Report of the quality standards subcommittee of the American Academy of Neurology and Child Neurology Society. *Neurology, 55,* 468–479.

Friedman, D. (2001). Employer supports for parents with young children. In Behrman, R. (Ed). *The future of children: Caring for infants and toddlers, 11*(1), 63–77.

geographyIQ.com. (2003). Rankings, population. Retrieved March 6, 2003, from www.geographyiq.com

Gillman, M., et al. (2001) Risk of overweight among adolescents who were breastfed as infants. *Journal of the American Medical Association, 285*(19), 2461–2467.

Glassbrenner, D. (2003). *The use of child restraints in 2002*. Washington, DC: National Center for Statistics and Analysis.

Halfon, N., et al. (in press). Summary statistics from the national survey of early childhood health, 2000. National Center for Health Statistics. *Vital Health Stat.*

Halfon, N., & Newacheck, P. (1999). Prevalence and impact of parent-reported disabling mental conditions among U.S. children. *Journal of the American Academy of Child and Adolescent Psychiatry, 38*(5), 600–609.

Health Resources Services Administration, Maternal and Child Health Bureau (2002). *Child health U.S.A. 2002*. Rockville, MD: Maternal and Child Health Information Resource Center, MCH00066.

Hebbeler, K., Wagner, M., Spiker, D., Scarborough, A., Simeonsson, R., & Collier, M. (2001). *National early intervention longitudinal study: A first look at the characteristics of children and families entering early intervention services*. Menlo Park, CA: SRI International.

Hodgkinson, H. (2001). Educational demographics: What teachers should know. *Educational Leadership, 58*(4). Retrieved February 6, 2003, from www.ased.org

Hoffman, C., & Wang, M. (2003). *Health insurance coverage in America: 2001 data update*. Washington, DC: The Kaiser Commission on Medicaid and the Uninsured.

Homes for the Homeless (2003). Fact sheet. Retrieved March 19, 2003, from www.homesforthehomeless.com/facts/html

Jain, A., Khoshnood, K., Lee, S., & Concato, J. (2001). Injury related infant death: The impact of race and birth weight. *Injury Prevention, 7*, 135–140.

Johnson-Green, E., & Custodero, J. (2002). The toddler top 40: Musical preferences of babies, toddlers, and their parents. *Zero to Three, 23*(1), 47–48.

Jones, N., & Smith, A. (2001). *The two or more races population: 2000*. Retrieved April 9, 2003, from www.census.gov

Kamerman, S. (1998). Child welfare and the under-threes: An overview. *Zero to Three, 19*(3), 1–7.

Kamerman, S. (2000). Early childhood education and care: An overview of developments in the OECD countries. Retrieved April 28, 2003, from www.childpolicy.org/kamerman.pdf

Kane, A., Mitchell, L., Craven, K., & Marsh, J. (1996) Observations on a recent increase in plagiocephaly without synostosis. *Pediatrics, 97*(6), 877–885.

Lamb, M. (1997). The development of father–infant relationships. In M. Lamb, (Ed). *The role of the father in child development*, (3rd ed.; pp. 104–120). New York: John Wiley & Sons.

Lee, S., Sills, M., & Oh, G. (2002). *Disabilities among children and mothers in low-income families*. Washington, DC: Institute for Women's Policy Research.

Lewis, C. (1997). Fathers and preschoolers. In M. E. Lamb (Ed.), *The role of the father in child development*. (3rd ed.; pp. 121–144) New York: John Wiley and Sons.

Lino, M. (2002) *Expenditures on children by families, 2001 annual report*. Alexandria, VA: U.S. Department of Agriculture, Center for Nutrition Policy and Promotion. Miscellaneous Publication No. 1528-2001.

Luby, J. (2000). Depression. In C. Zeannah (Ed). *Handbook of infant mental health* (pp. 382–296). New York: Guilford Press.

Madden, J., Soumerai, S., Liew, T., Mandl, K., Zhang, F., & Ross-Degnan, D. (2002). Effects of a law against early postpartum discharge on newborn follow-up, adverse events, and HMO expenditures. *New England Journal of Medicine 347*(25), 2031–2038.

March of Dimes (2001). *Data book for policy makers: Maternal, infant, and child health in the United States.* Washington, DC: Author.

March of Dimes and PriceWaterhouseCoopers (2002). *Newborn screening programs: An overview of costs and financing.* Washington, DC: Author.

Martin, J., Hamilton, B., Ventura, S., Menacker, F., & Park, M. (2002). Births: Final data for 2000. *National Vital Statistics Reports, 50*(5). Hyattsville, MD: National Center for Health Statistics.

Martin, J., Hamilton, B., Ventura, S., Menacker, F., Park, M., & Sutton, P. (2002). Births: Final data for 2001. *National Vital Statistics Reports, 50*(2). Hyattsville, MD: National Center for Health Statistics.

Martin, J., Park, M., & Sutton, P. (2002). Births: Preliminary data for 2001. *National Vital Statistics Report, 50*(10). Hyattsville, MD: National Center for Health Statistics.

Mather, M. (2000). The complex stories from census 2000 about America's diversity. Retrieved April 9, 2003, from www.prb.org

Mathews, T. (2001). Smoking during pregnancy in the 1990's. *National Vital Statistics Reports, 49*(7). Hyattsville, MD: National Center for Health Statistics.

McConnell, J. (1998, May–June). The joy of cloth diapers. *Mothering, 88*(42).

Military Family Resource Center. (2003). Overview of military child development system. Retrieved April 2, 2003, from http://mfrc.calib.com

Miniño, A. M., Arias, E., Kochanck, K. D., Murphy, S. L., & Smith, B. (2002). Deaths: Final data for 2000. *National Vital Statistics Report, 50*(15).

National Academy of Sciences. (2000). *Clearing the air: Asthma and indoor air exposures.* Washington, DC: National Academy Press.

National Association for Sport and Physical Education (2002). Early childhood physical activity guidelines. Retrieved March 31, 2003, from www.aahperd.org/naspe

National Center for Education Statistics (2002). Annual number of births: 1952 to 2012. Retrieved April 29, 2003, from http://nces.ed.gov/pubs2002/proj2012/table_b1.asp

National Center for Health Statistics. (2002). *Health, United States, 2002 with chart book on trends in the health of Americans.* Hyattsville, MD: Author.

National Center for Hearing Assessment and Management. (2003). Universal newborn hearing screening summary statistics. Retrieved March 15, 2003, from www.infanthearing.org

National Center for Injury Prevention and Control. (2000). U.S. homicide. Retrieved February 27, 2003, from www.cdc.gov/ncipc

National Coalition for the Homeless. (2002). Who is homeless? NCH Fact Sheet #3. Retrieved March 19, 2003, from www.nationalhomeless.org

National Highway Traffic Safety Administration. (2001). Traffic safety facts 2001: Children. Retrieved April 18, 2003, from www.nhtsa.gov

National Household Survey on Drug Abuse. (2001). Alcohol use. Retrieved April 23, 2003, from www.samhsa.gov/oas/nhsda

National Immunization Survey. (2001). Estimated vaccination coverage by coverage level and state. Retrieved February 24, 2003, from www.cdc.gov/nip/coverage/NIS/figures/01/01-4313.gif

National Institutes of Health. (2003). Higher SIDS risk found in infants placed in unaccustomed sleeping position. Retrieved March 17, 2003, from www.nih.gov/news/pr/feb2003/nichd-28.htm

National Organization on Fetal Alcohol Syndrome. (2003) What is fetal alcohol syndrome? Retrieved April 23, 2003, from www.nofas.org

National Institutes of Child Health and Development (NICHD) Early Child Care Research Network. (2001). Non-maternal care and family factors in early development: An overview of the NICHD Study of Early Child Care. *Applied Developmental Psychology, 22*, 457–492.

National Institutes of Child Health and Development (NICHD). (2003). Research on sudden infant death syndrome. Retrieved April 7, 2003, from www.nichd.nih.gov/about/women/health/sids_research.cfm

Nugent, K. (1991). Cultural and psychological influences on the father's role in infant development. *Journal of Marriage and the Family, 53*, 475–485.

Oser, C., & Cohen, J. (2003). *Improving early intervention: Using what we know about infants and toddlers with disabilities to reauthorize Part C of IDEA.* Washington, DC: ZERO TO THREE Policy Center.

Osofsky, J. (Ed.) (1997). *Children in a violent society.* New York: Guilford Press, 97–123.

Osofsky, J. (1999). The impact of violence on children. *The future of children: Domestic violence and children, 9*(3), 33–49.

Osofsky, J. (2000). Infants and violence: Prevention, intervention, and treatment. In J. Osofsky & H. Fitzgerald (Eds.). *WAIMH Handbook of infant mental health* (pp. 162–196). New York: John Wiley and Sons,

Osofsky, J., & Dickson, A. (2000). Treating traumatized children: The costs of delay. In J. Osofsky & E. Fenichel (Eds.) *Protecting children in violent environments: Building staff and community strengths.* Washington, DC: ZERO TO THREE.

Osofsky, J., & Fenichel, E. (2002). *Islands of safety: Assessing and treating young victims of violence.* Washington, DC: ZERO TO THREE.

Parrott, S., & Neuberger, Z. (2002). *States need more federal TANF funds.* Washington, DC: Center on Budget and Policy Priorities.

Paulsell, D., Nogales, R., and Cohen, J. (2003). *Quality child care for infants and toddlers: Case studies of three community strategies.* Washington, D.C.: ZERO TO THREE and Mathematica Policy Research, Inc.

Phillips, D., & Adams, G. (2001). Child care and our youngest children. In R. Behrman, (Ed.). *The future of children: Caring for infants and toddlers, 11*(1), 35–51.

Phillips, D., & Young, J. (2000). Birth weight, climate at birth and the risk of obesity in adult life. *International Journal of Obesity and Related Metabolic Disorders, 24*(3), 281–287.

Polk, D. (1997, May–June). For models of universal child care check out the (international) neighbors. *Children's Advocate,* Action Alliance for Children.

Pontius, K., et al. (2001). Back to sleep – tummy time to play. *PM&R Update, 4*(4).

Population Reference Bureau. (2002). Women of our world data sheet. Retrieved March 22, 2003, from www.prb.org

Population Reference Bureau. (2003a). A century of progress in U.S. infant and child survival. Retrieved March 23, 2003, from www.prb.org

Population Reference Bureau. (2003b). Quick facts. Retrieved March 17, 2003, from www.prb.or

Pruett, K. (2000). *Fatherneed: Why father care is as essential as mother care for your child.* New York: The Free Press.

Raco, A., Raimondi, J., DePonte, S., & Brunelli, A. (1999). Congenital torticollis association with craniosynostosis. *Child's Nervous System, 15*, 163–169.

RAND. (1998). The armed services' response to the military child care act. *RAND Research Brief.* Retrieved April 13, 2003, from www.rand.org/publications/RB/RB7521

RAND. (2003). The military child care act of 1989. Retrieved April 13, 2003, from www.rand.org/publications/R/R4145

Rivers, J. (2001). Mothers of all competency. Retrieved April 18, 2003, from www.nzcer.org.nz/whatsnew/rivers.htm

Rutherford, K. (2001). Shaken baby/shaken impact syndrome. Retrieved April 25, 2003, from http://kidshealth.org

Ryan, A., Wenjun, Z., & Acosta, A. (2002). Breast-feeding continues to increase into the new millennium. *Pediatrics, 110*, 1103–1109.

Schechter, D., Coates, S., & First, E. (2001). Observations of acute reactions of young children and their families to the World Trade Center attacks. *ZERO TO THREE, 22*(3), 9–13.

Schickedanz, J. (1999). *Much more than the ABCs: The early stages of reading and writing.* Washington, DC: National Association for the Education of Young Children.

Schieve, L., Jeng., G., Wilcox, L., & Reynolds, M. (2002). Use of assisted reproductive technology – United States, 1996 and 1998. Retrieved April 21, 2003, from www.cdc.gov/mmwr

Schmidley, D. (2003). The foreign-born population in the United States: March 2002. *Current Population Reports.* Washington, DC: U.S. Census Bureau.

Schulman, K. (2002). *The high cost of child care puts quality care out of reach for many families.* Washington, DC: Children's Defense Fund.

Shonkoff, J., & Phillips, D. (Eds.). (2000). *From neurons to neighborhoods: The science of early childhood development.* Washington, DC: National Academy Press.

Silver, G., & Pañares, R. (2000). *The health of homeless women: Information for state maternal and child health programs.* Baltimore: Johns Hopkins University, School of Public Health.

Smith, K. (2002). Who's minding the kids? Child care arrangements: Spring 1997. *Current Population Reports.* Washington, DC: U.S. Census Bureau, Household Economic Studies

Teitler, J. (2001). Father involvement, child health and maternal health behavior. *Children and Youth Services Review, 23*(4/5), 403–425.

The Children's Foundation (2002). *2002 Child care licensing study.* Washington, DC: Author.

Thompson, B. (in press). *2002 Department of Defense demographics report.* Arlington, VA: Military Family Resource Center.

Thompson, R.A. (2001). Development in the first years of life. Caring for infants and toddlers. *The Future of Children, 11*(1), 21–34.

United Nations Children's Fund. (2002). The state of the world's children, 2001. New York: Author.

United Nations Children's Fund (2003a). Breastfeeding and complementary feeding. Retrieved May 1, 2003, from www.childinfo.org/eddb/brfeed?current1.htm

United Nations Children's Fund (2003b). Immunization coverage. Retrieved June 2, 2003, from www.childinfo.org/eddb/immuni/leagafr.htm

United Nations Educational Scientific and Cultural Organization. (2002a). Social transformations and their implications for the global demand for early childhood care and education. *UNESCO Policy Briefs on Early Childhood, 8.*

United Nations Educational Scientific and Cultural Organization. (2002b). Women, work, and early childhood: The nexus in developed and developing countries. *Policy Brief 4.*

United Nations Population Division. (2003). World population prospects: The 2002 revision. Retrieved April 8, 2003, from www.un.org/esa/population

University Medical Center Tucson Arizona. (2003). Breastfeeding your baby. Retrieved February 20, 2003, from www.azumc.com/UMC

U.S. Bureau of Labor Statistics. (2001a). National compensation survey—child care workers. Retrieved March 7, 2003, from http://data.bls.gov

U.S. Bureau of Labor Statistics. (2001b). Single years of age—poverty status of people in 2000. Retrieved March 27, 2003, from http://ferret.bls.census.gov/macro/032001/pov/new23_005.htm

U.S. Census. (2000). Your gateway to Census 2000. Retrieved January 16, 2003, from www.census.gov/main/www/cen2000.html

U.S. Census Bureau. (2001). Households, by type, age of members, region of residence and age, race and Hispanic origin of householder, March 2000. Retrieved February 21, 2003, from http://www.census.gov/population/www/socdemo/hh-fam/p20-537_00.html

U.S. Census Bureau. (2002). Population estimates and projections. Retrieved November 13, 2002, from http://www.childstats.gov/ac2002/indicators.asp?iid=8&id=1

U.S. Conference of Mayors. (1998). The status report on hunger and homelessness in American cities—1998. Retrieved February 20, 2003, from www.usmayors.org/uscm/homelss/hhsummary/html

U.S. Department of Agriculture Economic Research Service (2001). Infant formula prices and availability: Final report to congress. Retrieved January 29, 2003, from www.ers.usda.gov/publications/efan02001

U.S. Department of Agriculture Food and Nutrition Service. (2002). WIC at a glance. Retrieved March 11, 2003, from www.fns.usda.gov/wic/programinfo

U.S. Department of Education. (1999). *Start early, finish strong: How to help every child become a reader.* Washington, DC: Author.

U.S. Department of Education. (2000). *Growing pains: The challenge of overcrowded schools is here to stay.* Washington, DC: Author.

U.S. Department of Education. (2001). *23rd annual report to Congress on the implementation of the Individuals with Disabilities Education Act.* Washington, DC: Author.

U.S. Department of Education, Office of Special Education Programs, Data Analysis System (2003). Part C data. Retrieved March 5, 2003, from www.ideadata.org/PartCdata.asp

U.S. Department of Health and Human Services. (1995) Disability among children. *ASPE Research Notes*, January. Retrieved February 18, 2003, from www.aspe.hhs.gov

U.S. Department of Health and Human Services. (2000a). *Healthy people 2010: Understanding and improving health.* (2nd ed.) Washington, DC: U.S. Government Printing Office.

U.S. Department of Health and Human Services. (2003). *Head Start program information report 2001–2002.* Washington, DC: DHHS, Head Start Bureau.

U.S. Department of Health and Human Services, Administration for Children and Families. (2002a). *Early Head Start information folder, 2002 EHS fact sheet.* Retrieved March 19, 2003, from www.acf.hhs.gov/programs/hsb/research/factsheets/02/hsfs.htm

U.S. Department of Health and Human Services, Administration for Children and Families. (2002b). Making a difference in the lives of infants and toddlers and their families: The impacts of Early Head Start. Washington, DC: Author.

U.S. Department of Health and Human Services, Administration for Children and Families. (2002c). The AFCARS report April 2000(3). Retrieved March 20, 2003, from www.acf.dhhs.gov/programs/cb/publications/afcars

U.S. Department of Health and Human Services, Administration for Children and Families. (2002d). *The AFCARS report, interim FY2000 estimates as of August, 2002.* Retrieved March 12, 2003, from www.acf.hhs.gov/programs/cb/publications/afcars/report7.pdf

U.S. Department of Health and Human Services, Administration for Children and Families. (2003a). *CCDF: percentage of children served by age group FFY 2001.* Retrieved April 11, 2003, from www.acf.hhs.gov/programs/ccb

U.S. Department of Health and Human Services, Administration for Children and Families. (2003b). *Research to practice: Child care.* Washington, DC: Author.

U.S. Department of Health and Human Services, Administration for Children and Families. (2003c). *Temporary Assistance to Needy Families program (TANF) 5th annual report to Congress.* Washington, DC: Author.

U.S. Department of Health and Human Services Centers for Medicare and Medicaid Services (2003). EPSDT data retrieved February 21, 2003, from http://cms.hhs.gov/medicaid/epsdt

U.S. Department of Health and Human Services, Office of the Assistant Secretary for Planning and Evaluation. (1998). *Trends in the well-being of America's children & youth.* Washington, DC: Author.

U.S. Department of Labor Current Population Survey. (2002). *Employment characteristics of families in 2001.* Retrieved April 29, 2003, from http://www.bls.gov/news.release/famee.t06htm.

U.S. Environmental Protection Agency. (2000). *America's children and the environment: A first view of available measures.* Retrieved March 6, 2003, from http://yosemite.epa.gov/ochp/ochpweb.nsf/content/ACE-Report.htm/$file/ACE-Report.pdf

U.S. Fire Administration. (2001). *Children and fire in the United States: 1994–1997.* Federal Emergency Management Agency. Retrieved April 27, 2003, from www.usfa.fema.gov

Vissing, Y. (1996). *Homeless children: Addressing the challenge in rural schools.* Retrieved April 22, 2003, from http://www.ericfacility.net/ericdigests/ed425046.html

Von Kries, R., et al. (1999). Breast feeding and obesity: Cross sectional study. *British Medical Journal, 319(*7203), 147–150.

Wetzstein, C. (2002). Foreign adoptions grow to record levels. Retrieved March 19, 2003, from www.washingtontimes.com/national/20021206-98822234.htm

Whitebrook, M., Sakai, L., Gerber, E., & Howes, C. (2001). *Then and now: Changes in child care staffing, 1994–2000.* Washington, DC: Center for the Child Care Workforce.

Wulczyn, F., & Hislop, K. (2002). Babies in foster care: The numbers call for attention. *Zero to Three Journal, (22)*4, 14–15.

Wulczyn, F., Hislop, K., & Harden, B. (2002). The placement of infants in foster care. *Infant Mental Health Journal, 23*(5), 454–475.

Wulczyn, F., Kogan, J., & Harden, B. (in press). Placement stability and movement trajectories. *Social Service Review.*

Yeargin-Allsopp, M., Rice, C., Karapurkar, T., Doernberg, N., Boyle, C., & Murphy, C. (2003). Prevalence of autism in a US metropolitan area. *Journal of the American Medical Association, 289*(1), 49–55.

ZERO TO THREE (2003). Definition of infant mental health. Retrieved March 6, 2003, from www.zerotothree.org

ZERO TO THREE Policy Center (2003). The national evaluation of Early Head Start: Early Head Start works. Washington, DC: Author.